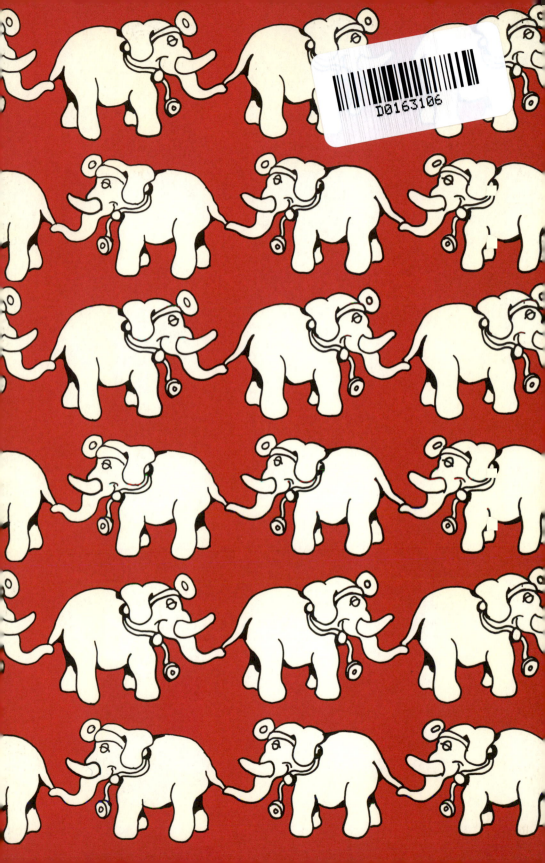

ELEPHANT MEDICINE
—AND MORE

ELEPHANT

—AND

MUSINGS OF

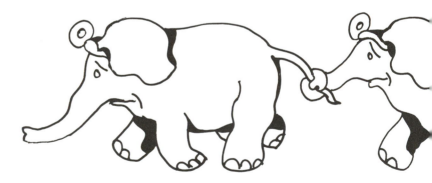

MEDICINE
MORE

A MEDICAL
EDUCATOR

Herbert L. Fred, M.D.

Educational Coordinator
HCA Center for Health Excellence
Houston, Texas

Formerly: Director of Medical Education
St. Joseph Hospital
Houston, Texas

MERCER
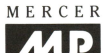

ISBN 0-86554-078-0

ELEPHANT MEDICINE
—AND MORE
Copyright © 1988
Mercer University Press
Macon, Georgia 31207
All rights reserved
Printed in the United States of America

∞ The paper used in this publication meets
the minimum requirements of American National
Standard for Information Sciences—Permanence
of Paper for Printed Library Materials, ANSI Z39.48-1984.

LIBRARY OF CONGRESS CATALOGING-IN-PUBLICATION DATA
Fred, Herbert L.
    Elephant medicine—and more: musings of a medical
        educator / Herbert L. Fred.
        181 pp.   15 x 23 cm.   6 x 9″
    Essays previously published in various sources.
    ISBN 0-86554-078-0 (alk. paper)
    1. Medicine—Miscellanea.   I. Title.
    [DNLM: 1. Education, Medicala—collected
works. 2. Ethics, Medical—collected works.
3. Nomenclature—collected works. 4. Professional
Practice—collected works. 5. Wit and Humor—
collected works.   WZ 7 F852e]
R708.F835   1988
610—dc19
DNLM/DLC   88-39602
for Library of Congress   CIP

CONTENTS

MEDICAL ETHICS   **126**

—AND MORE   **151**

*In loving memory
of my mother and dad,
Helen and Isie Fred*

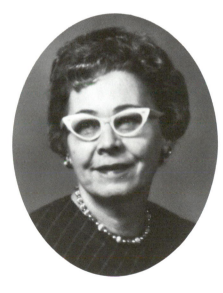

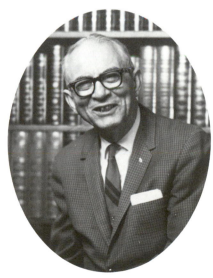

THE SPARROW'S EXAMPLE*

A horseman found a sparrow lying on his back in the middle of the road, feet up. When the horseman asked him why he was doing it, the sparrow said he'd been told the heavens were going to fall that day. The horseman laughed and asked him if he thought his puny little legs could hold the heavens up, and the sparrow replied, "One does what one can."

—ANONYMOUS

Saddened by society's growing attitude of indifference and by its diminishing quest for excellence, I applaud the sparrow. Each of us would do well to follow his example.

*Reprinted by permission from *St. Joseph Hospital Medical Surgical Journal* 1973; 8:187.

HOUSTON
C I T Y   M A G A Z I N E

BIG BUCKS
BIG BUILDINGS

JANUARY 1984 $1.75

THE 84 MOST INTERESTING PEOPLE OF 1984

The absolutely most choice of the choice

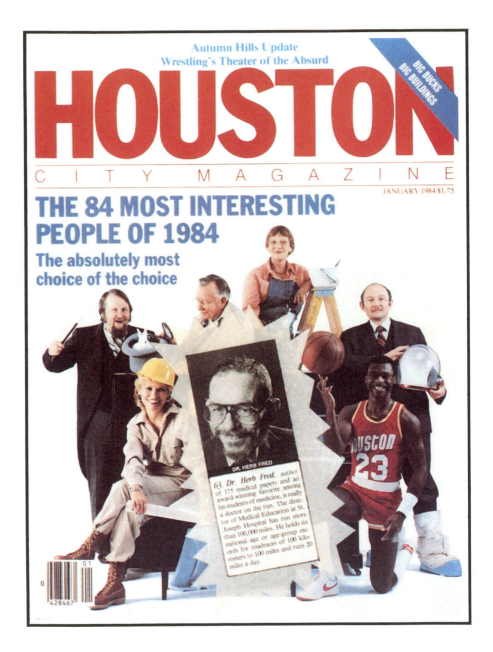

DR. HERB FRED

63. *Dr. Herb Fred*, author of 175 medical papers and an award-winning favorite among his students of medicine, is really a doctor on the run. The director of Medical Education at St. Joseph Hospital has run more than 100,000 miles. He holds six national age or age-group records for roadraces of 100 kilometers to 100 miles and runs 20 miles a day.

FOREWORD

Today, health-care professionals are writing more and more about more and more—which, in itself, is good. But they are writing less and less well—so poorly, in fact, that their products sometimes offend not only the sense but also the senses.

Elephant Medicine—and More is a happy exception to this trend. In this collection of witty and sage essays, Dr. Herbert L. Fred comments on the world of medical education, medical communication, medical practice, medical ethics, and more, often provoking a flash of recognition, a grin, or a moment of reflection. And this book shows that one can be a physician and still be a good writer.

"He is a card-carrying intellectual in the field of medicine with the ability to bridge the gap between the ivory tower and the real world of medical practice." So said a colleague who knows Herb Fred as a physician, teacher, administrator, writer, editor, and ultra-marathoner. Undoubtedly it was this wide range of interests and capabilities that prompted *Houston City* magazine to name Herb "one of Houston's eighty-four most interesting people in 1984." Each of these facets of his life is reflected in this book of essays.

After receiving a bachelor of arts degree from Rice Institute in Houston in 1950, Herb studied medicine at

Johns Hopkins University and received his M.D. in 1954.
He completed his internship and residency training at the
University of Utah Affiliated Hospitals in Salt Lake City.
Following two years in the U.S. Air Force, he returned to
the University of Utah as an instructor in medicine. In
1962 he went to Baylor College of Medicine in Houston as
an assistant professor of medicine. During his seven
years there, he was named the outstanding full-time
clinical faculty teacher by the senior classes of 1964 and
1965. In 1967 the seniors dedicated the Baylor annual, the
Aesculapian, to him.

In July 1969 he accepted the position of director of
medical education at St. Joseph Hospital, Houston, and in
1971 became a full professor of internal medicine at the
University of Texas Medical School at Houston. Between
1974 and 1979 the interns and residents at both the
UT Medical School and St. Joseph Hospital gave him a yearly
award for "Excellence in Teaching."

Throughout his teaching career, Herb has been a
visiting professor of medicine at numerous hospitals and
medical schools. In May 1984 he lectured at medical
colleges in Shanghai, Nanjing, and Xian in the People's
Republic of China.

In 1966, well before the current craze for physical
fitness, Herb became interested in developing a strong
body as well as a strong mind. Consequently, he began to
run. Starting with a win in a two-mile cross-country race,
he quickly graduated to marathons and then to
ultramarathons (100-kilometer, 100-mile, and 24-hour
races). From 1980 to 1983, he set a number of national
age and age-group records for ultradistances, including a
100-mile run in 17 hours, 2 minutes, 3 seconds at the age
of 53. Three years later he was still setting national age
records in 24-hour track runs. His interest and
participation in sports medicine led to his appointment

in 1979 as adjunct professor in the Department of Health and Physical Education at his alma mater, Rice University.

During this same period, Herb was writing extensively, at first on topics of clinical interest and then on his philosophy of medical education. To date, he has presented approximately 160 papers at scientific meetings and has published more than 200 articles in medical journals. He served on the editorial board of *Medicine and Science in Sports and Exercise* from 1979 to 1986 and has been on the editorial board of the *Annals of Sports Medicine* since 1982. In November 1984 he became editor-in-chief of *Houston Medical Journal.* That same year the American Osler Society recognized Herb's continued quest for quality in communication, teaching, and patient care by electing him to membership. Limited to seventy-five active members, the society recognizes and promotes the Oslerian ideals of a humanistic approach to the practice of medicine.

Every physician should read *Elephant Medicine—and More,* both for what it says and for the way it says it.
—*John P. McGovern, M.D., Sc.D., Litt.D.*

Dr. McGovern is the founder of the McGovern Allergy Clinic of Houston, Texas, the world's largest private allergy clinic. His fourteen faculty appointments include professorships in allergy and immunology, pediatrics, medical journalism, biomedical communications, and the history and philosophy of medicine at institutions such as Baylor College of Medicine in Houston, the University of Texas at Austin, the University of Texas Health Science Center at Houston, and the University of Texas Medical Branch at Galveston. He is also a fellow at Green College, Oxford University, in England.

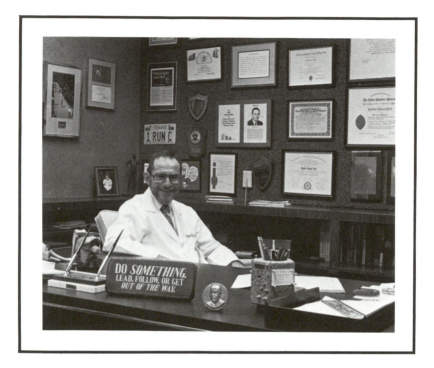

Herbert L. Fred, M.D.

PREFACE

As you will see, this book has little to do with elephants. It deals primarily with doctors who *act* like elephants.

In medicine, there's a saying: a general practitioner knows less and less about more and more until he knows nothing about everything, whereas a specialist knows more and more about less and less until he knows everything about nothing. Like most people, I know a little bit about a lot of things, but I don't know a lot about anything. So why this book?

Early in my medical career, I assumed that the more scientific articles I could write, the better doctor I'd be. One hundred fifty such articles later, I came to appreciate how much more there is to medicine than academics. Then, the focus of my writings changed, resulting in the essays assembled here.

The other major influence on these essays—as I now realize—was my father. He showed me that it's not what you *know,* but what you *do* that counts. A jeweler by trade, but above all a family man, Dad spent much of his adult life feeding and clothing the needy, arranging medical care for the indigent sick, and promoting goodwill between Gentiles and Jews, whites and blacks, rich and poor. I was immensely proud of him and loved him dearly.

On Dad's death in 1969, the editor of our hometown newspaper, the *Waco* (Texas) *News-Tribune,* wrote:

> The people whose lives were changed for the better by Isie Fred would fill a big football stadium if they all came together—and that is where Isie Fred would prefer to meet them. This community won't see the likes of him soon, if ever.
>
> Isie Fred's intense interest in his fellow human beings, his zest for living, his warm heart and his gift for action made him an unforgettable part of this community. He trailed laughter behind him like a cloud nearly always. His optimism was as contagious as the measles. Fortunate are those who shared life with Isadore Fred.

In retrospect, it was Dad's concern for others that led me into medicine, and for thirty years I have been a full-time medical educator. My job puts me in the classroom, in the laboratory, in the clinics, and at the patient's bedside. It brings me into daily contact with medical students, interns, resident physicians, private practitioners, and medical school faculty members. Under these circumstances, I have had ample opportunity to see how we doctors relate to each other and to our patients.

From my observations, I believe that most doctors work hard and mean well. But I also believe that doctors are a lot like elephants: we tend to follow the herd rather than think for ourselves. This mental inertia undermines patient care, dulls intellectual curiosity, impedes self-education, hinders decision making, and cripples effective communication. It is more common among doctors than alcoholism or drug abuse and is potentially more devastating to society. Yet it gets almost no attention.

In these essays, I have addressed this problem and related matters, offering solutions when I could.

The footnote splicing that readers will see here is not the attempt of the editor to mimic a surgeon's skill. Rather, it is an effort to render these articles—originally published in medical journals—more familiar to a university press readership. What I have crafted is an amalgam of both styles that should be acceptable to physicians as well as lay readers. It should also be noted that small-scale discretionary changes were made in transforming this series of previously published articles into a university press book. While the author has superlative self-critical instincts in his writing, some changes were made in the original texts—with regard to word choices, punctuation, and the like—in reissuing the articles in book form.

—ED.

ACKNOWLEDGMENTS

Special thanks are due Pat Robie and Mark Scheid for editorial assistance; Richard Blakely, Mary Scheid, and Ken Sack for reviewing the manuscripts; Geri Rochford for secretarial help; Adie Marks for the cartoons in the text; Glenn Knotts for encouragement; and the readers who responded to my work. I also appreciate the many medical students, house officers, academicians, and practicing physicians who inspired these musings.

My editor at Mercer University Press, Susan Carini, and Mercer's book designer and art director, Margaret Jordan Brown, have earned my highest respect and deepest gratitude. Their midwifery skills made delivery of this book exhilirating and almost pain-free.

Last, but foremost, I am indebted to my wife, Judy, for her unending patience and love.

MEDICAL EDUCATION

Crowded restaurants are common. How common are crowded libraries?

—H. L. F.
—in "Intellectual Anorexia"

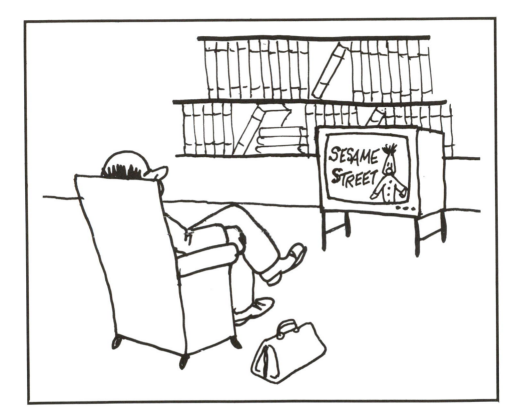

INTELLECTUAL ANOREXIA*

All wish to possess knowledge, but few, comparatively speaking, are willing to pay the price.

—JUVENAL
Satires 7†

An ever-spreading malady undermines our society. I call it intellectual anorexia. It typically strikes teenagers and young adults but endangers everyone. The victims demonstrate an attitude of indifference. They work strictly by the clock, have little pride, avoid sacrifice, shun competition, evade responsibility, and set few goals. Mediocrity is their norm. Cure requires restructuring of life-style and realignment of priorities. Specifically, those afflicted must feed their brains as methodically as they feed their stomachs.

Food for thought: Crowded restaurants are common. How common are crowded libraries?

---

*Reprinted by permission from the *Southern Medical Journal* 1975; 68:1468.

†Decimus Junius Juvenalis, Roman poet and satirist, c. A.D. 60-140.

WHAT'S THE DIFFERENCE . . .
AND WHAT DIFFERENCE DOES IT MAKE?*

A colleague received the following letter from his daughter:

Dear Dad,

It has been months since I left for college. Because I've been remiss in writing, I want to bring you up to date on matters. I'm getting along fine now. The skull fracture and concussion I got when I jumped out of the window of my dormitory when it caught on fire are pretty well healed. Fortunately, an attendant at the gas station near the dorm saw me jump. Since I had nowhere to live after the fire, he kindly invited me to share his basement room. He's a fine boy and we have fallen deeply in love and plan to get married. We haven't set the date yet, but it will be before my pregnancy begins to show. I know you'll welcome him even though he is of a different religion than ours.

Now that I've brought you up to date, I want to tell you that there was no dormitory fire; I didn't have a concussion or skull fracture; I am not pregnant; and there isn't any man in my life. Nevertheless, I am getting a *D* in History and an

---

*Reprinted by permission from the *Southern Medical Journal* 1980; 73:1559.

F in Algebra, and I wanted you to see those marks in their proper perspective.

Your loving daughter . . .

That letter points out what we all know but too frequently forget: there is more to an education than academics. With this in mind, I'd like to offer my perspective on the education of physicians in the customary medical school system contrasted with that in the private community hospital.

I recognize that this subject is controversial, but I feel qualified to address it. Teaching internal medicine to medical students and house officers has been my job for twenty-one years. For ten of those years I taught full-time in the medical school system. Then I became the full-time director of medical education at a large private community hospital, where I oversee a variety of residency training programs. This additional responsibility has necessarily broadened my view of education to encompass many specialties. Accordingly, my remarks apply in general to any of the clinical disciplines.

The Medical School System

Medical schools are set up to educate students, but the majority devote equal or greater attention to research. The teaching faculties consist largely of two groups: young fellows and instructors, fact-filled but experience-thin, and older professors, highly proficient in a narrow segment of their specialty. Both groups spend long hours lecturing, writing papers, working in the laboratory, or traveling to meetings. These priorities, whether school-decreed or self-imposed, limit contact between faculty and trainees.

Teaching, therefore, takes place more in the conference room than at the bedside. Consequently, students and house officers spend more and more time attending conferences and less and less time attending patients. Having little direct access to the teaching staff, they turn to house officers only one or two years their senior for much of their instruction. Complicating matters further, the case materials and milieus in city-county, federal, and university hospitals are not typical of those that most physicians encounter in their own practices. Finally, patients frequently become important not as people in need of help but as "diseases" linking education with research.

The Private Community Hospital

Here, good patient care is the first priority. Education is a close second and research third. These priorities focus attention more on the patient than on the disease. The majority of physicians who comprise the teaching faculty have been in private practice for many years. Free of rigorous academic commitments, virtually all of them are available to students and house officers for instruction on a one-to-one basis. Teaching by house officers is minimal. The case material and setting are those that most physicians meet in private practice.

Comment

These are the important differences I see between the two training systems. What difference do these differences make? The answer depends on what the individual plans to do. If his goals are mainly academic, the customary medical school system lacks sufficient "everyday" medicine to give his scientific pursuits practical direction. If his interests lie in the care of people, private community hospital training is invaluable. Yet good patient care does not just happen. It requires skillful use of continually updated scientific knowledge and methods. For that, the private community hospital with residency training programs needs a good working relationship with a medical school.

Thus, either system alone comes up short. Together they can supply the training doctors need.

THESE ARE THE DAYS*

These are the days when interns have reason to gripe. Unless they demonstrate unflagging commitment, interns are fired—they don't have formal contracts.

Their schedule is grueling. Daily work rounds with the ward resident, fellow intern, and chief nurse begin promptly at 7:00 A.M. These rounds, lasting two hours, are sacred; only a bona fide emergency can interrupt them. Often they take place again in the evening. Interns work every day and every other night. While on duty, they rarely find time to sleep. When off duty, they typically leave the hospital about 8:00 P.M., but never without reviewing problem cases with their colleagues on call.

Their duties seem endless. They start and maintain all intravenous therapy. Aided at times by the residents and medical students, they do all of the admission and follow-up blood counts, urinalyses, stool guaiac tests, sputum stains, skin tests, and electrocardiograms. They draw every blood sample for culture and make the stains and microscopic studies on every specimen of pleural, ascitic, spinal, pericardial, and joint fluid. They determine

---

*Reprinted by permission from the *Southern Medical Journal* 1979; 72:513-14.

urine and fecal urobilinogen levels, measure the 24-hour urine protein and glucose concentrations, and examine stools for ova and parasites. Those on night call draw the early-morning blood samples from about thirty patients. That task, undertaken with frustratingly blunt (nondisposable) needles and ill-fitting glass syringes, has to begin at 5:00 A.M. or earlier to be finished before work rounds. They fill out the requisition slips for all laboratory procedures and are responsible not only for recording the results in the patient's chart but also for reciting them on demand.

They have to squeeze in time for daily chart rounds. During this ritual, the intern and the resident scrutinize all in-patient records and correct any deficiencies they find. Good record keeping is an inviolate law. "A sloppy chart indicates a sloppy doctor," the professor says, and defective records invariably bring down his wrath on the offenders.

Interns and residents are speakers at weekly Grand Rounds. That assignment compels them to spend time in the medical library studying diseases in depth. In the process they learn how to research a topic, how to read with discrimination, and how to give a formal presentation to a discerning audience.

They must prepare vigorously for teaching rounds. After the intern and the resident select the case, they prime everyone involved, including the patient and his family. They make certain that the patient will be in his room, appropriately gowned, when the professor arrives and that a nurse will be in attendance. They bring the best literature on the subject to the conference room, where they outline on a blackboard the important case data. They have on hand all of the patient's past and current medical records; a microscope with which to examine relevant urine sediments, blood films, and tissue sections; and x-ray view boxes for display of pertinent roentgenograms. Case presentations have to be clear, concise, and well organized. Then the professor takes over.

Interns cannot substitute technology for either physical diagnosis or the need to think. Identifying mitral stenosis, for example, requires detection by thoughtful physical examination. Echocardiography is not possible. Diagnosing hypercalcemia requires thinking of it and then ordering a specific test for the serum calcium concentration. The sequential multiple analyzer (SMA) is not available.

These are the days when a constant bed shortage limits admissions to the very young, the very old, or the very sick. Moreover, no coronary-care or intensive-care units exist, and life-support equipment is crude. These circumstances obligate interns to monitor their patients, not with machines, but with frequent trips to the bedside and long beside vigils. They also attend every operation and witness every autopsy on their patients. From such routines they become proficient at physical diagnosis, learn the pathophysiology and natural history of disease, and understand when to treat and why.

These are the days when postgraduate medical training ingrains discipline, stimulates the taste for continual self-education, and creates mutual respect among all hospital personnel.

What days *are* these? The days twenty-five years ago when I was an intern in the main teaching hospital of a state university.

Since then, the internship has changed, though it remains a difficult year. But it *should* be, for nothing worthwhile comes easily. And practicing medicine well is both difficult and worthwhile.

LUCUBRATION
—AND THEN SOME*

As sheer casual reading matter, I still find the English dictionary the most interesting book in our language.
—ALBERT JAY NOCK
"Memoirs of a Superfluous Man"

I can never remember whether *cumulative* has one *m* or two. For the umpteenth time, I reached for my dictionary. It opened to the word *lucubration*. I had never heard of *lucubration,* so I read on. I learned that it stems from the Latin *lucubrare,* to work by lamplight, and from the basic word *lux,* or light. A further definition is "studied or pretentious ideas expressed in speech or writing." In that regard, I hope you won't call this essay a lucubration even though I did write it at night.

My curiosity kindled, I embarked on a search for other such pearls. I soon discovered *concinnity,* which sounded to me like *obscenity.* But concinnity denotes elegance of literary style in adaptation of parts to a whole or to each other. Thus, I would hope that my effort here displays concinnity.

---

*Reprinted by permission from the *Southern Medical Journal* 1986; 79:234.

Still on my intellectual scavenger hunt, I came across *grandiloquent.* I hope no one applies that term to this causerie. Regardless, the five minutes I had spent in the Land of Serendip was both entertaining and informative. And with a sense of satisfaction, I put the dictionary back on the shelf.

Then for the umpteenth time plus one, I wondered whether *cumulative* has one *m* or two.

RECOMMENDED READING*

In 1979 the estimated number of biomedical articles being published annually was two million, and the publication growth rate was increasing geometrically.[1] Keeping up, therefore, poses an obvious problem: you would have to read 5,500 articles a day to make sure you saw everything of relevance.[2]

I believe that being a competent doctor requires more than having the latest scientific facts. I also believe that some of the most rewarding information in medical journals has little to do with science per se. Four recent papers illustrate my point.

One offers a poignant and sobering reminder that all health-care professionals "are here to serve people, not machines, schools or computers."[3] It tells of an incident

---

*Reprinted by permission from *Houston Medical Journal* 1986; 2:119-20.

[1]Bernier CL, Yerkey AN: *Cogent Communication: Overcoming Information Overload.* Westport, CT, Greenwood Press, 1979, p. 39.

[2]Haynes RB, McKibbon KA, Fitzgerald D, et al.: How to keep up with the medical literature: I. Why try to keep up and how to get started. *Ann Intern Med* 105:149-53, 1986.

[3]Kashani IA: The reason for our profession (*Letter*). *West J Med* 145:247, 1986.

in which an individual's ego gets in the way of rendering expedient care to a dying patient. In a somewhat analogous article, a young house officer confesses to placing his own needs above those of his elderly, distraught patient.[4] I daresay all of us are guilty from time to time of such misdeeds. What good, then, is knowing the latest developments in our field if we lose sight of our mission?

In another paper, a psychiatrist fantasizes about his own obituary and the kind of posthumous company in which he might find himself.[5] He exposes the superficiality and dishonesty so common in human behavior, but does so with humor and grace. How many purely scientific reports leave you entertained as well as informed?

The fourth article traces entrepreneurship in medicine from the Greco-Roman era to the present.[6] It concludes that no absolute contradiction exists between the entrepreneurial spirit and the spirit of traditional medical ethics. Whether or not you agree with its conclusions, the article will enlighten you.

Recommended reading for students and practitioners of medicine does not ordinarily include references to the obligations of our profession, to our own frailties, to speculative thinking, or to medical history. It should!

---

[4]West A: Personal view. *Br Med J* 293:754, 1986.

[5]Wilkins R: Personal view. *Br Med J* 293:132, 1986.

[6]Jonsen AR: Ethics remain at the heart of medicine. Physicians and entrepreneurship. *West J Med* 144:480-83, 1986.

LEARNING MEDICINE*

*The physician's continuing education . . . is largely a
process within himself, one he pursues on his own. Most
of his true learning—the part that sticks with him—is what
he does for himself, by himself.*

—GEORGE T. HARRELL
J Med Educ 33:217, 1958

The year is 1954 and morning teaching rounds are in
progress at Salt Lake County General Hospital. I am an
intern and have just finished presenting the case of a
woman with unexplained splenomegaly to Dr. George
Cartwright, a renowned hematologist. My diagnosis is
lymphoma, but I mention hepatic cirrhosis, sarcoidosis,
amyloidosis, and brucellosis as possibilities.

Dr. Cartwright enjoys challenging and being
challenged by students and house officers. This day is
no exception. After examining the patient, he cocks an
eyebrow, smiles, and says smugly: "Herb, how long has
this woman had leprosy?" With that, he walks away,
announcing that he will return for a follow-up the next
day.

I am stunned. Did he find something I had overlooked,
or is he kidding? Had I really erred that badly? If so, what

---

*Reprinted by permission from the *Southern Medical Journal* 1988;
81:422-23.

will he think of me? And what will the medical students and other house officers think?

My self-doubt and my threatened ego spur me to prove that Dr. Cartwright is wrong and that I am right. Of course, I dare not challenge him without obtaining sufficient ammunition from the medical library. I have twenty-four hours to become an expert on leprosy.

After much reading and deliberation, and after questioning and examining the patient again, I decide that she doesn't have leprosy. When I inform Dr. Cartwright of my conclusion, he pats me on the shoulder, grins, and says, "You're right, Herb. She doesn't have leprosy. But you know a lot more about leprosy now than you did yesterday, don't you?"

Indeed I did! But I didn't know at the time that Dr. Cartwright was doing more than offering me an opportunity to broaden my knowledge. He was, in fact, testing my grit, my priorities, my intellectual curiosity. And he was prodding me to do what skilled clinicians often do: verify or redefine the problem, reexamine the patient, review the accumulated evidence, and scrutinize their own thinking.

Throughout high school, college, and medical school, I thought that learning depended on having a good teacher. When I was an intern, however, I began to realize that the most active role in my education belonged to me. Later, when I myself became a teacher, I realized that a good teacher teaches by promoting learning; and he promotes learning primarily by the questions he asks, not by the answers he gives. Repeated exposure to this Socratic method teaches the student the types of questions to ask himself and when to ask them. From then on he learns most and best from one teacher— himself.

Those who truly want to learn everything they can about medicine soon discover that there are no uninteresting patients. Dr. Max Wintrobe, department chairman during my postgraduate training, put it this way: "Any patient is potentially a textbook of medicine. If you read about and reflect on every symptom, sign, and laboratory finding that your patient displays, one thing will lead to another, and your learning will never end."

Take the patient with "stroke," for example, and ask yourself these questions. Is the main problem in or outside the head? Is it infectious, neoplastic, or traumatic? Is it embolic, thrombotic, or hemorrhagic? Does it involve arteries, veins, or neither? Is it cardiac, pulmonary, hepatic, or renal in origin? Does it relate to acid-base imbalance, fluid derangement, electrolyte disturbance, hormonal dysfunction, abnormal blood sugar, altered blood pressure, coagulation defect, seizure disorder, demyelinating process, degenerative disease, substance abuse, drug overdose, poisoning, or combinations thereof? How far and how fast should the work-up proceed? Can judicious therapy cure or ameliorate the condition?

Pondering questions such as these—questions that differ from patient to patient and from illness to illness—is part of what makes the practice of *good* medicine so time-consuming and difficult, yet so worthwhile. But without an ongoing effort to learn, a good practitioner inevitably becomes a mediocre practitioner—and a "stroke" is just a "stroke."

SINE QUA NONS
FOR THE COMPLEAT PHYSICIAN*

Twenty-two years ago I spoke before senior students at Baylor College of Medicine on what I considered to be "sine qua nons for the compleat physician." Though much in medicine has changed in the interim, the requisites I discussed then—hard work, striving for excellence, communicating effectively, intellectual honesty, and avoiding arrogance—remain applicable today. But today I am older and realize now what I failed to realize then: the compleat physician must also show compassion, common sense, and wisdom.

Hard Work

When I was an intern, a certain resident physician—currently chief of endocrinology at a university medical center—regularly one-upped me by quoting pertinent articles he had abstracted on cards. His knowledge and method of storing facts impressed me, so I asked to duplicate his cards. He refused, encouraging me instead to devise my own filing system. I did. Now, thirty-four

---

*Reprinted by permission from the *Southern Medical Journal* 1988; 81:883-84.

years later, I have one of the largest and most serviceable collections of medical reprints anywhere—all done without computers. And I continue to spend several hours daily, weekends included, keeping my files updated and functional. Hard work? Yes. But worth it, because routinely reviewing and collating material from 150 medical journals keeps me abreast of new developments, refreshes my memory on many aspects of medicine, and helps me teach.

Dr. William Bean, the Sir William Osler Professor of Medicine Emeritus at the University of Iowa College of Medicine, summarized it this way: "There is no magic vitamin, no capsule of intellectual chemotherapy, which will serve in the place of the one medicine which gives excellence—hard work."[1]

Striving for Excellence

My mentor, Dr. Max Wintrobe, an international authority on diseases of the blood, was never completely satisfied with his or anyone else's performance. He often said, "No matter how good a job we do, we can always do a better one."

Dr. Raymond Pruitt, former dean of the Mayo Graduate School of Medicine–Mayo Clinic, wrote: "Excellence, wherever sought, is not easily found. Its possession requires a mind quick to discernment of flaws, a nature intolerant of needless error, a will unbending in pursuit of high accomplishment."[2]

---

[1]Bean WB: A plea for excellence. *J Iowa State Med Soc* 40:22-24, 1950.

[2]Pruitt RD: On being almost right. *Cardiovasc Res Center Bull* 2:34, 1963.

Communicating Effectively

In talking with each other and with our patients, we frequently use a long, nonspecific word when a short, more precise one would be better. According to Bean,

> We say pathology when we mean lesion, though few say "how fine the astronomy!" when we admire the stars, or "how pleasant the horticulture!" when we look at a flower garden. . . . When we call for consultation, in our unconscious egomania, we say "have dermatology or orthopedics see him." There are a hundred other awkward word usages which are no clearer than the correct and usually simpler American idiom.[3]

Intellectual Honesty

A highly respected surgeon, Dr. Oscar Creech, Jr., once said:

> The phony exists in every vocation and has been vividly caricatured. Yet that which is comically ridiculous in other professions appears tragic when enacted by the physician. For he, more than any other man, finds his customers (the patients) completely at his mercy—they having placed themselves so deliberately. And when he distorts the facts of a case for his own rather than the patient's gain, he violates his exclusive position of trust.[4]

Dr. Creech also stated:

> None of us likes to appear ignorant nor do we enjoy being in error. The senior medical student feels that he must answer the questions of freshmen and sophomores or he

---

[3]Bean WB: A soliloquy for house officers. *J Student Am Med Assoc* 5:29-31, 1956.

[4]Creech O Jr: The voice of the cricket. *Bull Tulane Univ Med Faculty* 17:53-56, 1957.

isn't worthy of his high position. The senior resident, idol of medical students, interns and assistant residents, hesitates to say "I don't know" or "It was a mistake to operate on that patient" or "I completely missed the diagnosis," for he might quickly lose his following. Furthermore, weekly staff meetings would be painful affairs indeed. And so, a confused reply is given, an error in diagnosis rationalized, an operative mishap covered up. [And] the young physician ... has suddenly become aware that a mediocre performance can be made to appear first-rate if presented properly.[5]

Though dishonesty is sometimes a matter of interpretation, we should never condone it, particularly in medicine, because the results can be tragic.[6]

Avoiding Arrogance

An episode from the children's classic *Pinocchio* lucidly illustrates this theme.

Pinocchio has been hanged, and famous doctors of the realm—a crow, an owl, and a cricket—assemble to determine whether the puppet is dead or alive. The crow believes the puppet is already quite dead, but that if he isn't dead, it would be a sign that he is still alive. Next, the owl concludes that the puppet is still alive, but that if he isn't alive, it would be a sign that he is dead. Finally, the cricket, unimpressed by the performance of his fellow consultants, says, "In my opinion, the wisest thing a prudent doctor can do, when he doesn't know what he is talking about, is to be silent."[7]

---

[5]Ibid.

[6]Fred HL, Robie P: Dishonesty in medicine. *South Med J* 77:1221-22, 1984.

[7]Creech: Voice of the cricket.

Arrogance among physicians is common and understandable but lamentable. As a group, we are intelligent, have an inordinate amount of schooling and training, characteristically answer only to ourselves, and routinely render important decisions regarding the lives of our fellow human beings. Our patients, in turn, confer on us a superhuman power. No wonder we tend to be haughty, egocentric, omnipotent. Often, arrogance is a front for ignorance and will crumble as knowledge builds. Whatever the cause, we should fight any godlike tendency with an "anti-deiotic," a mixture of humility with honesty.

And finally, my coda—

Compassion, Common Sense, and Wisdom

These now top my list of sine qua nons. Why, then, did I exclude them from my original presentation? Because at that time I was too young to appreciate their importance.

Compassion can develop early if we have the right role models. When we witness compassion, we can give it more easily; but we cannot feel its full significance until we receive it when we need it. Though most physicians have compassion, many are unable to show it.

Common sense, in contrast to book sense, is inherent. We either have it or we don't. And not using it is worse than not having it.

Lastly, wisdom: If it comes at all, it comes with age.

To Max Wintrobe— Master Mentor*

Last September, while reminiscing with Dr. Wintrobe about my days as a house officer on his service, I learned that the November issue of this journal would be devoted to him. Unfortunately, the publication deadline prevented me from contributing to that issue. Hence this belated tribute to a great teacher.

To most physicians, the name Max Wintrobe means a long list of scientific publications and a classic textbook on hematology. To me, however, Max Wintrobe means much more.

I first met Dr. Wintrobe in June 1954, shortly before beginning my Straight Medical Internship in his department. I spent five years with him, four as house officer (including one as chief resident) and one as staff physician. The more I reflect on those years, the more apparent their value has become and the more my respect and admiration for Max Wintrobe have grown.

Dr. Wintrobe demanded much, both of himself and of those around him. He abhorred excuses, expected top effort, and rewarded only exceptional performance. He

---

*Reprinted by permission from *Medical Times* 1980; 108:23.

was always firm but always fair. He played no favorites and complimented or condemned colleagues just as rapidly and convincingly as he did the janitor or hospital administrator. He had the rare ability to criticize someone's work without making the individual feel personally attacked. He listened perceptively and spoke authoritatively, never leaving his audience in doubt as to where he and they stood, and why.

He rarely seemed satisfied. "No matter how good a job we do, we can always do a better one," he would say. Indeed, had I discovered the cure for leukemia, his response surely would have been, "That's fine, Herb, but why didn't you do that *last* year?"

Two additional statements he often made have stuck with me through the years. "If I do my job well, I'll never win a popularity contest." And, "I'd rather be respected than loved." Few, in fact, did love him, but all respected him.

His unwavering commitment to excellence was often traumatic. If the patient complained that the breakfast biscuits were cold, Dr. Wintrobe scolded the ward personnel. If the chest film was overexposed, he confronted the radiologist. If the case presentation was not crisp and well organized, the students and house staff felt his displeasure.

His effectiveness as a teacher was not as evident to me then as it is now. He used the Socratic method, asking many questions but supplying few answers. He strongly believed that one could learn much from *any* patient, regardless of how routine the case appeared. He would invariably discover something in the history or physical examination that others had missed or inappropriately ignored. He taught best, however, by setting examples, particularly the examples of hard work, self-discipline, self-education, clear thinking, intellectual honesty, and intellectual curiosity.

Although Dr. Wintrobe never wasted a moment at work, he knew when to relax and how to play. He was an avid skier, appreciated the fine arts, especially the symphony, and enjoyed travel. In contrast to his demeanor in the hospital, he was charming in his home. He and his wife, Becky, loved to entertain and were gracious hosts. Dinner with the Wintrobes was the social highlight of my training days.

Max Wintrobe has profoundly influenced countless students and house officers, giving their lives new impetus and direction. That is his finest and most durable contribution.

MEDICAL COMMUNICATION

Words form language, language enables communication, and communication is our link with each other. Without communication, marriages fail, businesses fold, and education flounders.

—H. L. F.
—in "Foreword, Forward, Four-Word, or Four-Ward?"

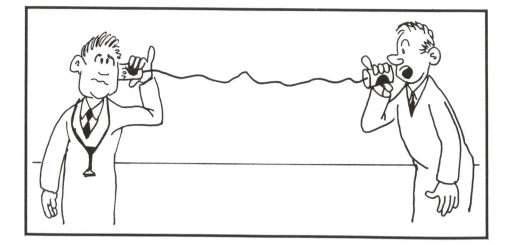

ATYPICAL CHEST PAIN:
A TYPICAL HUMPTY DUMPTY TERM*

"When I use a word," Humpty Dumpty said, in rather a scornful tone, "it means just what I choose it to mean— neither more nor less."

—LEWIS CARROLL
Through the Looking Glass, ch. 6

Like Humpty Dumpty, we doctors occasionally use a word to mean just what we choose it to mean, and we unwisely assume that everyone knows what we mean when we use it. A good example is our use of the word *atypical* to describe chest pain. Indeed, "atypical chest pain" is cropping up more and more in teaching conferences, in patients' records, in the medical literature, and in casual conversations throughout the hospital. Yet what does the term mean?

To answer this question, I went first to the medical library, where I found confusing and conflicting information. Some articles on chest pain used *atypical* in reference to clinical features atypical of angina

---

*Reprinted by permission from *Houston Medical Journal* 1986; 2:83-84.

pectoris.[1] Another used it to describe pain atypical of cardiac or esophageal origin.[2] Several articles mentioned "atypical chest pain" but didn't define it,[3] while one review didn't mention the term at all.[4]

Next, I asked fifty physicians—practicing internists and house officers in internal medicine—how they interpret or use the term *atypical chest pain.* About half of them said that atypical chest pain means atypical angina pectoris, but almost as many said that it means chest pain of unknown origin. One said that the term is meaningless. A few confessed to using it for an admitting diagnosis when they want to postpone further thought. A few others indicated that they diagnose "atypical chest pain" when they want to persuade a consultant to take over the patient's care or do a special procedure, such as coronary arteriography or esophagoscopy.

---

[1]Lee MG, Sullivan SN, Watson WC, Melendez LJ: Chest pain—esophageal, cardiac, or both? *Am J Gastroenterol* 80:320-24, 1985.

Levine HJ: Difficult problems in the diagnosis of chest pain. *Am Heart J* 100:108-18, 1980.

Channer KS, James MA, Papouchado M, Rees JR: Anxiety and depression in patients with chest pain referred for exercise testing. *Lancet* 2:820-23, 1985.

[2]Henderson RD, Wigle ED, Sample K, Marryatt G: Atypical chest pain of cardiac and esophageal origin. *Chest* 73:24-27, 1978.

[3]Bansal S, Toh SH, LaBresh KA: Chest pain as a presentation of reactive hypoglycemia. *Chest* 84:641-42, 1983.

Lee TH, Cook EF, Weisberg M, et al.: Acute chest pain in the emergency room: Identification and examination of low-risk patients. *Arch Intern Med* 145:65-69, 1985.

Greenwood RD: Mitral valve prolapse in childhood. *Hosp Practice,* August 15, 1986, pp. 41-44.

[4]Harrison TR: Clinical aspects of pain in the chest. *Am J Med Sci* 269:75-110, 1975.

Another point: whether chest pain is atypical or not depends on what we perceive as typical. Our perception of "typical," in turn, depends on the extent of our medical knowledge and on the time we spend evaluating the patient. Thus, the pain may be "atypical" of the manifestations that cluster near the top of the bell-shaped curve but "typical" of those on either slope of the curve. Or the pain may be truly "atypical" of the disease we are considering at the moment (e.g., angina pectoris) but clearly "typical" of one we aren't considering (e.g., pulmonary thromboembolism). And in our zeal to prove our initial impression, we may set in motion a "fruitless search for infallibility,"[5] which results in a multitude of ill-directed, expensive, time-consuming, and sometimes dangerous studies.

The practice of medicine is hard enough without using Humpty Dumpty terms. I suggest, therefore, that we dispose of the term *atypical chest pain.* Substituting *chest pain, ? cause*[6] or *unexplained chest pain* would reduce the risk of miscommunication, remind us of our ignorance, stimulate us to think, and keep us honest with ourselves and our patients.

———————

[5]Todd JW: Value of positive myocardial infarction imaging in coronary care units. *Br Med J* 1:690, 1979.

[6]Wilcox RG, Roland JM, Hampton JR: Prognosis of patients with "chest pain ? cause." *Br Med J* 282:431-33, 1981.

IDIOPATHIC*

When there is no explanation, they give it a name, which immediately explains everything.

—MARTIN H. FISHER,
as quoted by H. Fabing and R. Marr in *Fisherisms*

Idiopathic— Physicians repeatedly write it, read it, say it, and hear it, but we never seem to think about it. When I thought seriously about the word *idiopathic,* I decided that we should drop it from our vocabulary or change the way we spell it.

Idiopathic simply means "arising from an unknown cause." Thus, if a patient has unexplained bloody urine, we say that he has "idiopathic hematuria." If he has perplexing belly pain, we say that he has "idiopathic abdominalgia." If he has inexplicable convulsions, we say that he has "idiopathic epilepsy."

"Idiopathic" is a pseudoscientific and quasi-intellectual way of saying "I don't know." But since most doctors have difficulty saying "I don't know," the tag "idiopathic" is destined to remain forever ensconced in the medical lingo. This is unfortunate, because our habit of substituting labels for diagnoses all too frequently lulls

*Reprinted by permission from the *Southern Medical Journal* 1986; 79:351-52.

us into diagnostic complacency and dulls any further cerebration. The patient, in turn, suffers the consequences. To combat this ongoing danger, I have coined the term *idiotopathic.* It looks and sounds like *idiopathic,* but it makes us more mindful of our ignorance—while still satisfying our penchant for labels.

MUST*

"We all use words not only without knowing their true meaning but also without appreciating their *shades* of meaning."[1] A good example of this is *must,* a word flooding current scientific literature. *Must* usually connotes compulsion or force, inevitability or certainty. It leaves little or no alternative. If not used judiciously, however, *must* loses the desired effect and becomes imperialistic, amusing, or overwhelming. To wit, the following quotations from recently published medical articles:

"To this list MUST now be added internal pancreatic fistulas."

Comment: "Must is for kings."[2]

"I feel certain that there will not be a recurrence of the ulcerations, but the patient MUST follow my direction of maintaining heavy weight elastic stocking support."

---

*Reprinted by permission from the *Southern Medical Journal* 1977; 70:1392.

Patricia Robie is coauthor of this article.—ED.

[1]Paton A: How I write a paper. *Br Med J* 2:1115-17, 1976.

[2]Dekker T, Chettle H: *Patient Grissil* 4:1603.

Comment: "We physicians tend to be an egotistical lot."[3]

"We all MUST continue to strive for the best approach and leave our prejudices behind."

Comment: We must also love motherhood, apple pie, and the flag.

"The search MUST continue for improvements in colon cleansing."

Comment: The search must continue, too, for cleaner medical writing.

"Torsion of the greater omentum, therefore, MUST be added to the list of differential diagnoses when one is considering peptic ulcer disease."

Comment: Oh, come on now . . .

"Renal involvement MUST be exceedingly rare, since we found only three reported cases."

Comment: And if it's Tuesday, this must be Belgium. Finally, two mega-"musts":

"Three problems MUST be solved before ultrasound mammography can be used as a screening device: First, additional clinical data MUST be accumulated. Second, the number of ultrasonograms needed for diagnosis MUST be reduced. Third, special equipment designed for ultrasound mammography MUST be developed."

"We, as professionals, MUST address these problems. We MUST calculate benefits carefully, we MUST assiduously collect data on risks, and we MUST set a fair price for services rendered. All of this we MUST do."

Comment: Whew!

Conclusion: We must use *must* meticulously. Yes, we MUST . . . MUST . . . MUST . . .

---

[3]Mathis JL: You must play God almost every day. *Hosp Phys* 3:21, 1973.

To My Knowledge*

"To my knowledge" is a phrase whose appearance in current medical literature has reached epidemic proportions. Why? Does any writer know everything about his topic? Does the ploy shield the author from criticism and excuse him from more work? Does the device improve a manuscript's clarity, ensure its validity, or strengthen its message? Does the tactic satisfy discerning readers?

No. Well, perhaps not. At least, not to my knowledge!

---

*Reprinted by permission from the *Southern Medical Journal* 1976; 69:1455.

IS IT BILE OR BILIRUBIN?*

From time to time there appear articles that make a plea for greater specificity in speaking and writing.[1] This is as it should be, since precision in the communication of knowledge is important to the progress of science. In line with this thesis, we shall point out reasons for abandoning the inappropriate use of "bile in the urine," a phrase long entrenched in medical tradition.

Exactly how or when this phrase became common jargon is not certain. As early as 400 B.C. Hippocrates described jaundice and mentioned dark urine.[2] In the thirteenth century John Actuarius wrote that discolored urine resulted from admixture with bile, or more rarely,

---

*Reprinted by permission from *Archives of Internal Medicine* 1963; 111:405-406.

[1]Bean, WB: Tower of Babel 1961. *Arch Intern Med* 108:4-7, 1961.

Bean, WB: Tower of Babel 1962. *Arch Intern Med* 110:375-81, 1962.

[2]Adams, F: *The Genuine Works of Hippocrates.* Baltimore, William Wood & Company (division of Williams & Wilkins Company), 1929, vol. 1, p. 324.

with blood.[3] Richard Bright, in an excellent treatise on jaundice published in 1836, referred to the urine of his patients as being "highly tinged with bile" or "loaded with bile."[4] In 1845 Scherer isolated a crude preparation of biliverdin from icteric urine.[5] Further understanding of the bile pigments was facilitated by Heintz, who isolated bilirubin in 1851.[6] Since that time our knowledge of bilirubin metabolism has increased significantly.[7] Yet, despite twentieth-century information, there still persist nineteenth-century malapropisms such as "the urine was positive for bile."

There can be no excuse for perpetuating semantic confusion between bile and bilirubin. It should be obvious that bile contains many substances, only one of which is bilirubin. Furthermore, in patients with intra- or extrahepatic biliary obstruction, it is not the total secretion of the liver that is poured into the urinary tract, but rather the various conjugates of the pigment bilirubin. Indeed, in the presence of jaundice, it is these

---

[3]Mettler, CC: *History of Medicine,* edited by F. A. Mettler. Philadelphia, Blakiston Company (division of McGraw-Hill Book Company, Inc.), 1947, p. 293.

[4]Bright, R: Observations on jaundice: More particularly on that form of the disease which accompanies the diffused inflammation of the substance of the liver. *Guy Hosp Rep* 1:604-37, 1836.

[5]Gray, CH: *The Bile Pigments.* London, Methuen & Co., Ltd., 1953, p. xi.

[6]Castiglioni, A: *A History of Medicine,* translated and edited by E. B. Krumbhaar, 2d ed. New York, Alfred A. Knopf, 1947, p. 782.

[7]Schmid, R: *Metabolic Basis of Inherited Disease,* edited by J. B. Stanbury et al. New York, McGraw-Hill Book Company, Inc., 1960, pp. 226-70.

Billing, BH, Lathe, GH: Bilirubin metabolism in jaundice. *Amer J Med* 24:111-21, 1958.

conjugates—not bile—that color the urine and are detected by the routine laboratory methods. How, then, can one logically make a statement such as "The urine contains bile"? The retort "We all know what it means, so what difference does it make?" does not suffice, because it rationalizes into acceptance a physiologic inaccuracy.

Presumably, actual bile in the urine could result only from a direct communication between functioning biliary and urinary tracts. Although this situation has been produced experimentally in dogs by anastomosing the common bile duct to the proximal end of the ureter,[8] we are aware of no evidence that bile ever has been found in the urine of man. This is regrettable, because such a case might afford an opportunity for one to announce, "The bile was positive for urine!"

The authors do not expect these remarks to bring about an en masse switch from "bile in the urine" to the preferred "bilirubinuria." Nevertheless, we do hope that the foregoing will encourage some medical students, house officers, clinicians, academicians, and members of editorial boards of scientific journals to be more precise when recounting the urinary findings of jaundiced patients.

—John M. Eiband, M.D.
—Herbert L. Fred, M.D.

Department of Internal Medicine
Baylor University College of Medicine

---

[8]Pearce, RM, Eisenbrey, AB: A method of excluding bile from the intestine without external fistula. *Amer J Physiol* 32:417-26, 1913.

FOREWORD, FORWARD, FOUR-WORD, OR FOUR-WARD?*

From time to time the English language poses problems for even the most educated among us. As an example, take the word *foreword.* Notice how much it sounds like *forward, four-word,* and *four-ward* and how similar the spellings of these words are. The resemblances end here, however.

Foreword, a noun, refers to prefatory comments (as for a book or journal), especially when written by someone other than the author. *Forward* is an adjective, noun, adverb, or transitive verb, depending on its use. Thus, "The boy who was so forward became the team's forward and moved forward whenever he would forward the ball." *Four-word* and *four-ward* are adjectives, as in "a four-word phrase" and "a four-ward area."

Now, let's go a step further. Compare "The fire gutted a four-ward area" with "The fire gutted a forward area." These sentences sound alike, look much alike, and are grammatically correct, but they convey different thoughts because *four-ward* and *forward* have different

---

*Reprinted by permission from the *Medical Journal of St. Joseph Hospital* 1983; 18:179-80.

meanings. Misusing, misspelling, or mispronouncing just one word can misinform or confuse the reader (or listener, as the case may be).

Why all this fuss about words? Because words form language, language enables communication, and communication is our link with each other. Without communication, marriages fail, businesses fold, and education flounders.

In its continuing efforts to keep education from floundering, the *Medical Journal* devotes this entire issue to medical education. Immediately after this foreword, Bar-Sela takes us backward— back, in fact, to antiquity— as he eruditely discusses the beginnings of medical education. Girard then brings us up to the late nineteenth century with a delightful essay on the birth of Osler's textbook of medicine. Next, Myers leads us forward to artificial intelligence and authoritatively demonstrates a type of computer program certain to receive major emphasis in tomorrow's educational arena.

On matters more current, Scheid effectively addresses the glaring need for good communication between physicians and patients. Moser appropriately reminds us that the key to continuing medical education is *self-education*. Hawes laments the failure of medical school and residency training to prepare him adequately for private practice. Wollangk warns that court decisions and government regulations are placing ever-increasing constraints on the delivery of health care. And Taylor describes an innovative role for college students in cancer research.

For each of these contributions and for the help of Mrs. Pat Robie, I close this foreword by putting forward a four-word "Thank you, very much."

ABBRS*

"He's got a CA and is SOB," the consultant says to the intern as they leave Intensive Care.

The patient's son, listening intently nearby, becomes irate: "I don't know what CA means, but you have no business calling *my* dad an SOB!"

"You misunderstand," the consultant replies. "We often don't have time to spell everything out. CA refers to cardiac arrhythmia, and SOB stands for short of breath."

This incident occurred in my hospital, but I suspect it could have occurred just as easily in yours. In fact, if my experience is any gauge, no hospital is immune.

Like the consultant I quoted, we tend to forget that the only person who invariably knows what an abbreviation stands for is the one who uses it. I, for example, would have interpreted CA to mean cancer. Yet, a book on medical arcana lists fifty *additional* definitions for CA; it also offers four definitions for SOB, excluding the colloquial one.[1] While this text will delight the

---

*Reprinted by permission from the *Southern Medical Journal* 1987; 80:1339.

[1]Logan CM, Rice MK: *Logan's Medical and Scientific Abbreviations.* Philadelphia, JB Lippincott, 1987.

abbreviationado and acronymnist in all of us, it drives
home the point that abbreviations, especially in
medicine, have myriad meanings. And deciphering any
abbreviation depends primarily on our frame of
reference.

Consider BE. I'm an internist, and in my mind BE
stands for barium enema. But some infectious disease
specialists use BE for bacterial endocarditis; pathologists,
for Barrett's esophagus; neurologists, for brain edema;
and orthopedists, for below the elbow.

Even seemingly unambiguous abbreviations can
mislead. BM is not always a bowel movement; it
frequently refers to black male. Moreover, the
hematologist may think of BM as bone marrow, the
endocrinologist as basal metabolism, and the pathologist
as basement membrane. Similarly, PND is not necessarily
paroxysmal nocturnal dyspnea. It may signify postnasal
drip to the otolaryngologist, partial neck dissection to the
surgeon, and postneonatal death to the pediatrician. And
what about AS? To me it denotes aortic stenosis; to many
it indicates arteriosclerosis. Others associate AS with
Anglo-Saxon, anxiety state, atrial septum, Adams-Stokes,
or atropine sulfate.

Because of their ambiguity, abbreviations in medicine
can be dangerous. If they go unquestioned, particularly in
doctors' orders and prescriptions, the patient may get the
wrong test or the wrong medication, with devastating
results. Almost every doctor, nurse, and pharmacist can
recall a mishap of this sort.

Why do we abbreviate so much? Because
abbreviating is part of the macho of being a doctor. And
because it saves time—except for those who have to
crack our code.

Can we halt this pandemic? Only when we value
clarity and precision over self-serving, thoughtless

shortcuts. Only when we concede that our abbreviations can do nothing for patients but place them at increased risk: emotional, financial, and physical. Then, it's simple—D.A.!

SCHOLARLY*

Don't appear so scholarly, pray. Humanize your talk, and speak to be understood.

—MOLIÈRE, 1663
The Critique of the School for Wives

Have you ever had a manuscript rejected for publication because it was too short? I have. And each time, the word *scholarly* was involved. The following story typifies these experiences.

You have spent a lot of time preparing your article. To make sure that your message comes through clearly, you have conscientiously culled all superfluity from the final copy. Then, with high hopes, you mail it. Weeks pass. At last, the editor responds: "I regret to inform you that we cannot accept your paper. You haven't developed your topic in sufficient detail or depth." What he won't say in his letter of rejection—but may admit when pressed—is: "Your paper isn't scholarly enough. It doesn't comment on every ramification of your topic, and it lacks the provocative theorizing characteristic of learned presentations. In short, it's too short!"

*Reprinted by permission from the *Southern Medical Journal* 1988; 81:909.

In academia, *scholarly* is a word we use frequently. But what does it really mean? When I asked that question of erudite people, their answers varied considerably. This didn't surprise me, because according to *Webster's Ninth New Collegiate Dictionary,* the definition of *scholarly* is implicit at best: "of, characteristic of, or suitable to learned persons: learned, academic."

Thus, "scholarly," like beauty, is in the eye of the beholder. And like so many other words in the English language, it is a Humpty Dumpty term:

> "When I use a word," Humpty Dumpty said, in rather a scornful tone, "it means just what I choose it to mean—neither more nor less."[1]

Scholarly is also a buzzword, one that we wield to impress our subordinates and to compliment or denigrate the work of our colleagues. And, in the publishing game, this role of "scholarly" can sink, or save, a manuscript.

Some journal editors and commercial publishers—even some university presses—opt for bulk over brevity, size over substance, matter over mind. If everyone used this logic, however, manuscripts without padding and puffery wouldn't qualify as "scholarly" and might not merit publication. And the Ten Commandments, Declaration of Independence, and Gettysburg Address—each pithy, perspicuous, and profound—might never have made it into print.

---

[1]Lewis Carroll: *Through the Looking Glass,* ch. 6.

Dizzy Medical Writing*

After completing his glorious pitching career, Dizzy Dean became a popular baseball announcer. In response to a listener who accused him of not knowing the King's English, Dizzy said, "Old Diz knows the King's English. And not only that. I also know the Queen is English."

Old Diz may have known the King's English, but you couldn't prove it by how he spoke. Similarly, many physicians and scientists may know the King's English, but you couldn't prove it by how they write. We decided, therefore, to present the 1983 "Dizzy Awards" for outstandingly dizzy medical writing. Only recent articles in prominent American medical journals were eligible.

The winners are:

The Postponed Because of Wet Grounds Award

"The presence of a bladder tumor in our patient, and in previous reports, demonstrates again . . ."

—We are saddened to learn that the medical literature, in addition to its many other ailments, now has bladder tumors.

---

*Reprinted by permission from the *Southern Medical Journal* 1983; 76:1165-66.

Patricia Robie is coauthor of this article.—Ed.

The No Runs, No Hits, Two Errors Award

"Until such a determination is made, physicians should inform their patients as to what the research to date do and do not show ..."
—Well, what *do* it show?

The Base on Balls Award

"During life use of the penis ..."
—Did ya hear about the guy who died, but ... ?

The Cases at the Bat Award

"Ninety of 360 patients had mild itching on admission and showed the same survival as the 249 nonitching cases."
—How would an itching case scratch itself, anyway?

The Triple Play Award

"The leiomyoma was lost to follow-up, the saphenous vein leiomyosarcoma survived nine years, and the leiomyosarcoma of the IVC is six months without recurrence."
—So much for the tumors. But what about the patients?

The Out in Left Field Award

"Alpha factor analysis has been shown to yield a lower bound estimate to the number of factors and allow psychometric inference to a universe of variables."
—Take me to your leader.

The Balk Award

"Because of such incongruous findings between stipulated metabolic properties of muscle fiber types and maximum isometric strength and fatigability, the present investigation related fiber type composition with maximum isometric strength and fatigability of the plantar flexors using the same power and endurance subjects previously studied on knee extension strength."

—How's that again?

The Signs from the Coach Award

"If we conceptualize IMV and SIMV in this way, we may be prompted to describe CPAP as IMV (or SIMV) + PEEP at an IMV (or SIMV) rate of zero. In fact, it is not uncommon to convert a patient from IMV/SIMV to CPAP by initially placing the patient on IMV or SIMV with PEEP and subsequently decreasing the IMV/SIMV rate in stepwise fashion to zero."

—Break this code and receive a year's supply of IUDs or a membership in the PTA.

The Extra Innings Award

"Subsequent to submission for publication, an additional seven patients have been treated."

—Always treat patients *before* submitting them for publication.

The Peanuts and Cracker Jack Award

"One case of anaphylaxis associated with both the ingestion of shrimp and exercise has recently been reported."

—Try eating the exercise an hour before the shrimp.

The Round-Tripper Award

"The presence of the glucagon sequence in the dominating forms of the enteroglucagons makes them an important source of glucagon."

—This is where I came in.

The Called on Account of Darkness Award

"The wide clinical spectrum of the lymphoproliferative diseases has excited interest and controversy for a century and there is no shortage of case histories that may be used by the protagonists to support, on the one hand, the view that there is a continuous gradation of conditions from the highly malignant metastasizing sarcomas of focal origin to the most benign form of Waldenström's macroglobulinemia, and, on the other hand, the view that there are multiple distinct entities which are confused with one another or appear falsely to show a continuous spectrum of merging forms because of superficial similarities resulting from the fact that all lymphoproliferative conditions arise in the same system of cells."

—Z Z Z Z Z Z Z

DIZZY MEDICAL WRITING: PART II*

Last year in this journal, we presented the first "Dizzy Awards" for dizzy medical writing. We named these awards in remembrance of Dizzy Dean and his unique use of the language while broadcasting baseball games. Since then—and without even trying—we have found so many new candidates that additional awards are necessary. The competition this time was so stiff that ties occurred in several categories.

The current winners are:

The Brought Up from the Minors Award

"In the present review nine patients were born and lived for many years in the 'calcific areas' of South Africa."

—There was an old woman who lived in a review . . .

The Caught Out of Position Award

"A palliative, noncurative, relief of symptoms has been reported in women with rheumatoid arthritis taking

---

*Reprinted by permission from the *Southern Medical Journal* 1984; 77:755-56.

Patricia Robie is coauthor of this article.—ED.

the oral contraceptive Enovid, a combination of progesterone and estrogen, by several investigators."

—This sentence was voted to be a prime example of the perils of the passive voice, by us.

The Switch Hitter Award

"The importance of classification is academic since none to date can handle all of the described anomalous possibilities."

—Anomalous possibilities are definitely harder to handle than possible anomalies.

The Time Called Award (a tie)

"Although rare, this form of secondary syphilis has been reported in the past."

and

"Cholesterol pericarditis with mildly elevated or normal pericardial cholesterol content has been reported in the past."

—To date, has either of these findings been reported in the future?

The Batted Out of Order Award

"Despite their profound inhibitory effect on both acid secretion and symptoms, all patients with the exception of those with proven metastases or the MEN type I syndrome underwent laparotomy to exclude a resectable lesion."

—Do these patients come in liquid or tablet form?

The Placed on the Disabled List Award

"The author experienced severe pulmonary edema after standard CPR in 20 of 71 patients who suffered sudden, unexpected cardiac arrest and regained heart function by CPR."

—Presumably, the author's severe pulmonary edema resolved.

The Wrong Ball Park Award (three-way tie)

"Infection caused by this organism has not been described outside the vascular system."
—Making this description *inside* the vascular system must have entailed an incredible voyage.

and

"Cardiac involvement, which is extremely rare in GD, has been described mainly in the pericardium."
—On which pages of the pericardium did the descriptions appear?

and

"Subsequently, most cases have been reported in menstruating women."
—Doesn't anyone report in journals anymore?

The Bag of Soda Pop and Cup of Hot Dog Award (a tie)

"Furthermore, unlike patients with nongonococcal bacterial arthritis, the results of blood and synovial fluid cultures are almost never concurrently positive in disseminated gonococcal infection."
— Patients, with or without arthritis, are *always* different from results.

and

"In contrast to the rat, the rate of gluconeogenesis from glycerol in man is too low to make a major contribution. . . . "
—We smell a rate.

The Debris on the Playing Field Award

"The studies were first subjected to a low pass temporal filtering technique which appends the temporally smoothed images to a file containing the unsmoothed data as well."

—We usually consign such unsmoothed prose to the circular file.

The Long Fly to the Pitcher Award (a tie)

"The acquisition of new observations makes it appropriate for us to re-evaluate our existing knowledge base and to make such modifications as are necessary to form a reasonably coherent theoretical whole."

—In short, knowledge begets knowledge.

and

" . . . she experienced a rapidly fatal outcome."

—In short, she died.

The Improper Gesture Award

"To the present time, behavioral investigations in sport settings have included a number of attempts to improve athletic performance by training coaches to manipulate reinforcement contingencies."

—Wouldn't it be more socially acceptable to reinforce contingent manipulations?

The Make-up Game Award (a tie)

"The role of the congested prostate in infertilogenesis is presented."

—Neologically speaking, the author of that statement need not worry about infertility.

and

"The conclusions from the present work, drawn from systematic protocolized gathering of data . . ."

—Questionologically speaking, are protocolized data gathered through a protocoloscope?

The Slow Roller Award

"The respiratory frequency was gradually decreased and the inspired minute volume gradually increased, in response to a sequence of arterial gas measurements, until after 30 min it could be established that, at a respiratory frequency of 72 b.p.m. with an I:E ratio of $\frac{1}{2}$ and an inspired minute volume of 3 litre min $^{-1}$, the peak airway pressure could be maintained in the range of 20-23 cm H_2O, and the arterial gas tensions with $F_{I_{O_2}}$ 0.6, were: pH 7.33 unit, PCO_2 5.8kPa, PO_2 11.5kPa."
—We must have made a wrong turn somewhere.

The Bad Hop Award

"It is a bit disturbing to note reports of women taking excessive doses of the tanning pills sold in Europe who have experienced amenorrhea."
—It is also a bit disturbing to read articles of writers submitting their findings to medical journals in America who dangle clauses like this.

The Blooper Award

"Usually (although invariably) HS is associated with venous insufficiency of the lower extremities."
—Huh?

The No Hitter Award

"The results demonstrated the absence of clinical evidence in all cases."
—As Shakespeare might have said, "nothing ado about nothing."

The Word Series Award

"The interdependence of anatomic systems, symbolic activity, and the external social and physical environment entails a holistic orientation and encourages interdisciplinary collaboration."

—The verbiage collector obviously didn't come by today.

The Batty Title Award (three-way tie)

"Training for Cross Country Skiing and Iron Status"

—Training for iron status is easier.

and

"Indwelling Urinary Catheter Infections in Small Community Hospital"

—What antibiotic is best for an infected hospital?

and

"Delayed Solitary Metastasis to the Radius of Renal-Cell Carcinoma"

—Was the carcinoma's "humorous" also involved?

The Breaking Pitch Award

"This case of spontaneous rupture of the external iliac vein may have been caused by thrombosis of the vein in the patient's pneumonia."

—If so, the treatment of choice would have been pneumonectomy.

The Peanuts and Cracker Jack Award

"Eight boiled shrimp with ketchup preceded the first bout of urticaria."

—. . . followed, no doubt, by a partridge in a pear tree.

DIZZY MEDICAL WRITING: CONCLUDED*

This is our third and last presentation of the Dizzy Awards—awards created to honor the late Dizzy Dean and given for excellence in bewildering, unintentionally comical, or just plain terrible medical writing. The winners, as before,[1] are excerpts from articles in prominent medical journals.

The Batty Title Award (four-way tie)

"Early Gastric Cancer in a United States Hospital"
—Presumably the hospital's chief complaint was pain in the middle of the corridor at the level of the ninth floor.

and

"Bacteremia in a Long-term Care Facility"

---

*Reprinted by permission from the *Southern Medical Journal* 1985; 78:1498-1501.

Patricia Robie is coauthor of this article.—ED.

[1]Fred HL, Robie P: Dizzy medical writing. *South Med J* 76:1165-66, 1983.

Fred HL, Robie P: Dizzy medical writing: Part II. *South Med J* 77:755-56, 1984.

—Did the organisms enter through the front or back door?

and

"Stability of Prevalence"

—Your guess is as good as mine.

and

"Training Effect in Elderly Patients with Coronary Artery Disease on Beta Adrenergic Blocking Drugs"

—Are trained drugs more effective than untrained drugs?

The Touch Every Base Award

"Alternatively, and in our view, far more likely, it is possible that if edema forms during the obstruction, it may be roentgenologically masked, perhaps by increases in lung volume."

—Would you care to qualify that statement?

The Switch Hitter Award

"Swingle et al reported 11 cases of left-sided inversion of 16,000 hospital admissions during one year."

—We always invert our hospital admissions to the right.

The Flagpole Award

"The common practice of misdiagnosing deep vein thrombosis clinically should be abandoned."

—Agreed.

The Safe All Around Award

" . . . unproductive diagnostic measures are unnecessary."

—Agreed.

The "It Ain't Over Til It's Over" Award (a tie)

"Very obviously, mouse connective tissue is not necessarily human connective tissue."
—Very obviously.

and

"Shock never developed if the disease was not serious."
— Seriously?

The Out in Left Field Award

"However, none of the subjects indicated any localized muscle pain or soreness of the delayed type at these times that they experienced later."
—We, however, wish to indicate diffuse pain and soreness of the immediate type brought about at this time by the statement above that we experienced earlier.

The Thirst Base Award

"For heat-acclimated subjects, we observed a hemoconcentration when hypohydrated."
—Never make research observations when you're hypohydrated.

The Blind Umpire Award

"Both eyes were quiet."
—Did the ears see anything?

The Cases at the Bat Award (three-way tie)

"Eight other cases obtained from liver biopsies referred from other hospitals were also reviewed."
—Did you hear about the alcoholic whose liver biopsy revealed a case of Scotch?

and

"Cases also smoked significantly more cigarettes than controls."

—Our cases smoke only when the record room is on fire.

and

"The cases, who were 20 to 49 years old at the time of diagnosis . . ."

—Our twenty- to forty-nine-year-old cases are either in cobwebs or on microfilm.

The Knot-Hole Award

"Subsequent reports suggest that colonoscopy can recognize angiodysplasia."

—But only after they've known each other for a long time.

The New Pitch Award

"The adult male and female predicted values for D_{LCO} and D_L/V_A were obtained from . . ."

—We know that sex has value, but we didn't know that values have sex.

The Wrong Pitch Award

"In only three patients did the urticaria subside coincident with treatment and clearing of the abnormal sinus roentgenogram."

—What treatment did you use for the roentgenogram?

The Signs from the Coach Award (three-way tie)

"This study in patients with IBS, PUD, and IBD and a previous one in nonpatients are the first to systematically and prospectively address themselves to PF."

—BS.

and

"Patients with type 2 or 3 of PSS, especially form A, carry a higher risk of developing severe LI than circumscribed scleroderma, type 1, or form B patients."

—Hand me the code book, Sam.

and

"At both the first and second study, the SS (or RR) correlated with the hepatic removal of sulfur colloid (ER_{SC}: r $= -0.59$; p < 0.001; HC_{SC}: r $= -0.56$; p $= 0.003$) and ICG (ER_{ICG}: r -0.85; p < 0.001; K_{ICG}: r $= -0.83$; p < 0.001). ER_{SC} correlated with ER_{ICG} (r $= 0.76$; p < 0.007) and both correlated with SS and RR consistent with intrahepatic shunting as the mechanism of decreased hepatic clearance and of sulfur colloid redistribution."

—*%#&$$!!*!!

The Final Out Award

" . . . in the remaining patients in whom ventricular fibrillation occurred without an associated myocardial infarction recurrence of sudden death is up to 40% within the first year."

—We thought only cats had nine lives.

The Batted Out of Order Award (six-way tie)

"After being discharged from the hospital, abdominal pain and the myxedematous features cleared and the effusions completely resorbed."

—Was the pain ambulatory when it left the hospital?

and

"If found incidentally, a complete workup should be performed."

—Has anyone seen a stray workup?

and

"While preparing a revision of the present case report, two additional cases of emetine myopathy were published."

—Write on.

and

"Although potentially lethal, close observation . . . can allow for necessary medical or surgical intervention."

—We're dying to get a good look, anyway.

and

"Commenting that most previous cases were managed with nephrectomy, a plea for renal repair or heminephrectomy is made."

—When a plea speaks, everybody listens.

and

"As a published novelist and former editor, rejection is not unfamiliar to me."

—Have you read "I Was a Former Editor" by Rejection?

The Who's on First, What's on Second Award

"We prefer to inject our patients in the face-down position."

—Doesn't that lead to a highly personal relationship?

The No Hits, No Runs, One Error Award (four-way tie)

"The nutrients delivered to the absorptive surfaces is determined by the gastric emptying rate."

—Are that so?

and

"The rate of contractions in different patients range from 60 to 200/min. . . "

—Home, home on the ranges.

and

"No vaccines will be useful, however, unless it is used."

—Vaccines is good for you.

and

"The causality of the coffee-lipoprotein relationships are not proved by these cross-sectional associations."
—Isn't they?

The Soda Pop Award

"It could be that coffee and tea drinkers who suffer symptoms of anxiety stop drinking it."
—Try drinking caffeine-free anxiety.

The Removed from the Lineup Award

"Two patients thought to be resectable after the above evaluations were found to be unresectable at laparotomy."
—Lucky for them.

The In-the-Hole Award

"Although they are frequently the centre of doctors' jokes, this report emphasizes the serious side to rectal foreign bodies."
—Although they are frequently the basis of bad writing, this sentence has a dangling modifier.

The Mechanical Pitcher Award (a tie)

"Table I collects the head and neck cases from these series."
—If you sit at *that* table, hold on to your hat!
and
"Femoral and radial artery catheters inserted by our protocol had a low incidence of catheter-associated infections."
—Evidently your protocol scrubbed up between cases.

The Game Plan Award

"The patient was treated with an epiglottis protocol."

—Was that protocol proprietary or generic?

The Bag of Soda Pop Award (three-way tie)

"Physical findings were different from two previous series originating in the United States."
—Regardless of their point of origin, series are always different from physical findings.

and

"Unlike routine overhead oblique views, at fluoroscopy the radiologist can determine the precise degree of obliquity needed."
—But some radiologists *are* oblique, at least in routine views.

and

"Grossly and microscopically, our patient's heart, similar to previous reports, showed petechial hemorrhage throughout. . . ."
—Such sentence structure would make any heart bleed.

The Squeeze Play Award

"In 21 studies on 18 patients, *in vitro* labeling of RBC was performed by injecting intravenously a commercially available kit containing 1 mg stannous chloride, 1 mg pyrophosphate, and 20 mg sodium triphosphate, diluted in 3 ml sterile saline."
—You injected the *whole* kit and caboodle?

The Balk Award

"However, in the absence of a thyroid primary, in view of the ability of carcinoids to form various polypeptide hormones (Milhaud *et al.,* 1974) (although not usually as much as was formed by Sweeney, McDonnell and O'Brien's tumour), and the finding of small amounts of amyloid in both our cases, Sweeney, McDonnell and O'Brien's case may be another carcinoid of the larynx forming an unusually large amount of polypeptide hormone and, secondarily to that, large amounts of amyloid."

—We disagree, we think.

The Word Series Award

"The striking results that have been achieved in the prevention and treatment of tetanus in developed countries and which can be achieved in developing countries also, are the result of the laboratory work of the preclinical scientists, namely, the anatomist, the biochemist, the physiologist, the microbiologist, the pathologist, the immunologist, the pharmacologist and their co-workers and of the clinical endeavors of the epidemiologist, the family physician, the internist and his subspecialty associates, the pediatrician, the surgeon and his subspecialty colleagues and the anesthesiologist."

—And what about the butcher, the baker, and the candlestick maker?

The Questionable Call Award

"Pseudotumor cerebri is a rare disorder occurring in the reproductive age range of females, thus occurring infrequently in pregnancy."

—And if it's Tuesday, this must be Belgium.

The Debris on the Playing Field Award

"Although effusions have been infrequently reported with benign mesothelial proliferation with effusion, ascites, pleural effusion, and/or pericardial effusion occurred in all of our patients."

—Multiple effusions equal confusion (and grammatical contusion).

The Make-up Game Award (a tie)

"The operationalization of group cohesion in sport research has suffered the same problems that plague the psychological literature."
—Indeed, neologismization plagues the entire scientific literature.

and

"On the other hand, when e.g. popliteal aneurysms thrombotize, they can destroy the peripheral circulation due to embolization."
—Thrombotizing aneurysms are also hard on our language.

The Bad Bounce Award

"Gardnerella vaginalis—not long ago, we called it Haemophilus vaginalis and dismissed it as a harmless commensal of the vaginal flora—but today, this fastidious bacterium has both a new name and a newly recognized potential to act as a pathogen in women and men alike."
—We wish this writer were as fastidious as the bacterium he describes.

The Placed on the Disabled List Award

"A physician at this time prescribed acetaminophen with codeine and cephalexin, most of which he subsequently vomited."
—The physician who treats himself has a fool for a patient.

The Caught Napping Award

"A CT scan of the brain, performed after the administration of sedation . . ."
—Wouldn't you really rather administer a sedative?

The Spring Training Award

"We encountered a case of right internal mammary artery to innominate vein fistula following subclavian vein catheterization and the projection of the coil spring was projected after transcatheter intravascular coil occlusion."

—We tried "in vein" to project meaning into this statement.

The Ball 5, Strike 4 Award

"Since regional lymph nodes rarely if ever metastasize . . ."

—Under the spreading lymph node tree . . .

The Died on Third Award

"It appears that if unrecognized, and if specific therapy is not instituted, mortality is universal."

—We recognize mortality and are eager to learn of your specific therapy.

The Blooper Award

"The value of the routine chest film in the patient with penetrating thoracic trauma cannot be underestimated."

—Oh yes it can!

And finally—

The Dean of Dizzies Award (a tie)

"The raw data were analyzed by means of alpha and canonical factor analytic techniques with varimax orthogonal rotation procedures used to place the underlying factor structures into interpretable positions."

—We interpret the position all right; it's the meaning that presents a problem.

and

"Thus, it appears that a broader conceptualization of cohesion which delineates the meaning of the construct as it relates to sport teams is needed (Carron, 1982), along with the development of operational measures which reflect cohesion as a multidimensional, rather than unidimensional, construct."

—???

Epilogue:

We draw two conclusions, one happy and one sad: The memory of Old Diz will be around for a long, long time. And so will dizzy medical writing.

MEDICAL PRACTICE

Physicians . . . do not have the privilege of shirking responsibility.

—H. L. F.
—in "Passing the Buck"

When the right diagnostic bell doesn't ring, you may be in the wrong belfry.

—H. L. F.
—in "When the Bell Doesn't Ring"

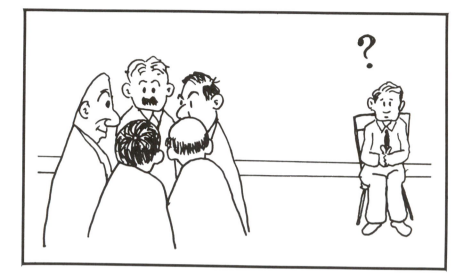

ELEPHANT MEDICINE*

From time to time almost all of us practice what I call "elephant medicine." Like elephants in the circus ring—the trunk of one holding on to the tail of the other—we plod mindlessly along, following without question the diagnoses and decisions of our colleagues. Sadly, in this parade, the patient gets run over.

Examples of elephant medicine abound. Here are a few:

● An asymptomatic man with a long history of smoking has a routine chest film that shows an irregular 2 x 2 cm mass in the right lower lobe. Five years earlier he had been treated at another local hospital for what he referred to as pneumonia. His physician now suspects lung cancer and orders cytologic examination of the sputum; the results are negative. Consultation with a pulmonary specialist leads to bronchoscopy and transbronchial biopsy, both of which disclose no abnormality. A thoracic surgeon then sees the patient and urges thoracotomy. The operation unveils an old pulmonary infarct.

---

*Reprinted by permission from the *Southern Medical Journal* 1981; 74:135.

Everyone followed the same line of thought: lung lesion—smoker—cancer. No one reviewed the records from the other hospital or examined the previous chest films. Had they done so, they would have found a diagnosis of pulmonary infarction and a chest film at discharge essentially identical to the current one. This oversight cost the patient part of his lung and a lot of his pocketbook.

• A seventy-nine-year-old man's only complaint is progressive weakness of three months' duration. On examination he is pale, but otherwise normal. His hematocrit value is 25 ml/100 ml and his total leukocyte count is 5,000/cu mm. Assuming that anemia of this magnitude in an elderly person most likely stems from gastrointestinal bleeding, his physician requests radiologic investigation of the entire alimentary tract. When these studies give normal results, a gastroenterologist performs proctosigmoidoscopy, colonoscopy, and esophagogastroscopy. These examinations also uncover no abnormality. At this point, someone finally directs attention to the patient's peripheral blood film. The erythrocytes are normocytic and normochromic, not microcytic and hypochromic as one would expect with chronic intestinal bleeding. More important, a few of the leukocytes are diagnostic of myelomonocytic leukemia.

The physicians automatically followed the dictum that anemia in elderly people most commonly reflects gastrointestinal bleeding. Their assumption precipitated costly and potentially debilitating examinations of the patient's alimentary tract when a critical interpretation of his peripheral blood film would have identified his real disease.

• A former movie actress has had unexplained fever for four years. During that time, she had gone to many physicians in different cities, submitting on each occasion to virtually the same diagnostic procedures and receiving the same types of treatment, all to no avail. On examination she is thin, talkative, and tense, and smokes cigarettes constantly. Other findings, including routine laboratory tests, are normal. Because the story suggests factitious disease, the patient is watched and is soon caught putting the lighted end of her cigarette to the thermometer.

Every time this woman consulted a physician, her "fever" triggered the same response—an array of referrals, a myriad of tests, and a multitude of therapeutic trials. Four years passed before someone put the case in perspective and stopped the medical merry-go-round.

In each of these cases, the physicians were well trained and well intentioned. Yet they all made the same mistake: they didn't think for themselves. They simply followed the herd.

PRESS BOX VISION*

Like football coaches, we physicians try to call the right play at the right time. To do so, we need what I call "press box vision"—a view of the situation in perspective. Coaches can get it relayed from the top of the stands; witness their earphones. For physicians, however, getting and maintaining perspective is much tougher. It takes a special blend of empathy, honesty, and book sense used with common sense.

Without press box vision, the coach and his team may lose. But football is just a game. Practicing medicine isn't.

H. L. F.

This editorial by Dr. Fred prompted a response from Mark R. Johnson, M.D., editor-in-chief, Oklahoma State Medical Journal.

---

*Reprinted by permission from *Oklahoma State Medical Association Journal* 1978; 71:153.

ON PLAYING DOCTOR

Well now, Dr. Fred, I'm sure you know that football *isn't* just a game with some people. Especially for some Oklahomans, Texans, Nebraskans, and Arkansawyers. It is, to paraphrase a famous football coach, not just a part of life. It is the only life.

And lately, it seems that practicing medicine *is* becoming a game, but one in which both teams as well as all the spectators will be losers. There will be no winners, even though everyone in the stadium, including the players, officials, and water boys will be bankrupting themselves making donations to support the game.

You and I don't practice medicine as if we were playing a game. However, if we were realists, I wonder if we would. Our senators and congressmen, our president and members of his cabinet have been playing doctor for so long and have had so much fun doing it that they have organized hundreds of laymen and put them on committees and councils and commissions that are authorized to play doctor with them. The game plan, which is proceeding as designed, is to take all the authority away from real doctors and give it to the play doctors. None of the responsibility or accountability is transferred, you understand; just the authority.

All rules and regulations that control this game of practicing medicine are now written in Washington by people who love to play doctor. The rules are changed regularly and whimsically by the self-appointed officials who never bother to ask for advice or guidance. The object of the game is no longer to achieve the goal of economical, high-quality health care: It is to defame and paralyze real doctors, substitute play doctors, and achieve the goal of total socialism.

I'm not sure that the game is football. Maybe it's button-button or Russian roulette. But it sure looks like a game to me.

M. R. J.

PASSING THE BUCK*

A number of card games that were formerly popular employed a token, or "buck," to indicate the dealer. After a hand was played, it was customary to pass the buck to the next player in order to prevent a mistake as to position of the deal. Considerable responsibility fell upon the dealer, since his wager determined whether the jackpot would be large or small. Consequently, timid players hesitated to deal. They were given the privilege of passing the buck when it came to them.

From this custom "passing the buck" came to stand for any method of evading responsibility.[1]

Everyone passes the buck from time to time. It is, in fact, so common that people tend to shrug it off as part of human nature. But in the health-care setting, where it pervades all ranks of personnel, passing the buck can be time-consuming and have expensive and even lethal consequences. This essay focuses on passing the buck as

---

*Reprinted by permission from the *Southern Medical Journal* 1982; 75:1164-65.

[1]Garrison WB: *Why You Say It.* New York and Nashville, Abingdon Press, 1955, p. 121.

I have observed it among certain attending physicians, consultants, and house officers in teaching hospitals.

Manifestations. These are numerous. They vary according to the physician's role in the case, but any form of passing the buck can appear in any member of the three groups.

Among *attending physicians,* the most obvious manifestation is failure to take charge. Faced with a busy schedule, fearful of being sued for missing something, and contending that their patients want it and deserve it, they order a myriad of tests and prescribe a multitude of drugs, hoping to detect and alleviate every conceivable ill. If the patient's condition does not improve or if the result of a test is abnormal, the attending defers to an army of consultants who march in and take over, each managing a part of the body. The process goes on and on until a definitive diagnosis surfaces, the patient's complaints subside, the patient or his family intervenes, or the patient dies. Throughout all this activity, the attending is but a spectator, watching a medical merry-go-round.

Among *consultants,* the most conspicuous manifestation is failure to stop the referring physician's buck. Although ideally positioned to halt the medical merry-go-round, they ride it instead, usually with gimmick in hand. Even when they know their gimmick is not indicated, they use it because "that's what the referring physician requested," "it's important for research," or "it's the only way to know for sure."

Among *house officers,* the manifestations are more diverse. Common is the attitude "I'm not really in charge, so why should I get involved?" Or, "The attendings have more experience than I do, so their way must be better." Another tactic is passive-aggressive behavior. They ignore the attending's written or verbal suggestions; they do not answer their beepers, later asserting, "I guess the battery was dead"; or they habitually miss or come late to conferences, alleging that they "got tied up." A third ploy is the "It's not back yet" response. When quizzed about the latest total leukocyte count or chest roentgenogram, they reply "It's not back yet," thinking that this statement exonerates them from tracking down such information.

Associated with all of these manifestations is a lack of useful communication among the physicians involved. The attendings' excuse is that house officers are so hard to find when needed that "it isn't worth the effort to locate them," and, when located, "They argue and ask too many questions." House officers, in turn, claim that attendings are hard to find, too, especially at night and on weekends. Moreover, they say that attendings, once contacted, frequently berate them, disagree with their proposed management of the case, or prevent them from gaining firsthand experience with a variety of diagnostic and therapeutic technics. They also maintain that the attendings are too often research-oriented, inflexible in their approach, not interested in teaching, not conversant with the medical literature, or not familiar with the patients they admit. So why communicate with them?

Communication with the consultant characteristically is indirect and impersonal, seldom face to face. A nurse or ward clerk is the messenger for orders such as "Have Dr. Smith see patient," or "Surgery consult, stat!" To make things worse, the consultant's communication with the referring physician is frequently a scribble on the patient's chart. In any event, the referring physician, be he attending or house officer, rarely takes issue with the consultant, presumably because it might make both of them uncomfortable; it would be politically unwise; or the consultant, as an expert, "must be right."

Ramifications. Attending physicians and *consultants* who pass the buck compromise their integrity and, without realizing it, lose the respect of their discerning colleagues. *House officers* who pass the buck hamper their own education by forfeiting opportunities to be active and influential in case management. As a consequence, they will become the buck-passing practitioners of tomorrow. Furthermore, their resentment toward attending physicians, along with the strained relationships that follow, hinder patient care.

And what about *the patient?* To him, passing the buck means literally passing bucks to his doctors and the hospital. Ordinarily, he is unaware that the number of bucks he passes relates directly to the amount of buck passing his doctors do. But if his doctors do enough buck passing, even the most trusting of patients will catch on. When that happens, the patient becomes angry and dissatisfied. At best, he forgives; at worst, he sues.

Management. The first step for those afflicted is to be honest: honest with their patients, honest with their associates, and honest with themselves. Having accomplished that, ...

Attending physicians should understand that *they* bear the responsibility for their patients' care, regardless of who does what. They should order tests and consultations to verify, not formulate, impressions.

Consultants should restrain themselves from taking charge of the case and from overusing their gimmicks. They should remember that they are mainly opinion givers, not decision makers.

House officers should be mindful of the ethical, moral, and legal perspectives of the private practitioner. They should appreciate that all patients have teaching value, including those they perceive as "dumps." And they should realize that there is more to education than academics—that the most active role in their education belongs to them, not to their teachers.

All of these physicians should work toward communicating effectively with one another. The attending physicians should notify house officers of impending admissions and discuss with them the purpose of hospitalization, the tentative diagnoses, and the therapeutic plans. Then they should insist that the house officers keep them informed of developments in each case. They should encourage them to express their views and should handle differences of opinion courteously. They should be willing to learn from as well as to teach house officers. Attendings also should talk with their consultants, telling them the precise reasons for the consultation.

Consultants, in turn, should speak directly with the referring physician, detailing their findings and explaining their recommendations. They should not rely on nurses, other doctors, or the patient to do that for them.

House officers should recognize that questions and ideas presented tactfully can secure cooperation from the most threatened of attendings and consultants.

Finally, physicians, unlike the timid card players of years past, do not have the privilege of shirking responsibility. For them, to quote President Harry Truman, "The buck stops here."

GIMMICKS*

*The patient may well be safer with a physician who is
naturally wise than with one who is artificially learned.*

—SIR THEODORE FOX
Lancet 2:801, 1965

Sales gimmicks are expected, and we all recognize
and accept them. Indeed, "new and improved" products
appear daily, each touted to solve another of life's
problems. Gimmicks in medicine are also common and
have been with us for years—from the flim-flam man of
years past hawking cure-alls off the back of his wagon to
the magazine ads of today promising surefire ways to
grow hair and melt fat.

Legitimate medical practice has its gimmicks, too.
They are technologically advanced, scientifically sound
procedures *misused* by physicians who are ill-trained,
ill-informed, lacking in self-confidence, looking for
shortcuts, fearful of litigation, or just plain greedy. Such
gimmicks are used without regard for their indications or
limitations and take precedence over diagnostic methods
that are simpler, less expensive, and equally effective.

---

*Reprinted by permission from the *Southern Medical Journal* 1983;
76:953.

Patricia Robie is coauthor of this article.—ED.

The current crop of potential medical gimmicks includes endoscopy for almost every orifice, computerized axial tomography, radioisotope scanning, ultrasonography, echocardiography, exercise stress tests, and coronary arteriography. These sophisticated techniques unquestionably enhance patient management—so long as the information they provide is interpreted cautiously and in relation to the findings from history, physical examination, and conventional laboratory studies.

Overreliance on modern technology is undermining the physician's use of his mind and five senses for diagnoses. Jumping from the patient's chief complaint to a host of tests and procedures is commonplace. And when that approach does not work, the physician simply orders more tests or seeks consultation. This malady of practice is making the skilled clinical diagnostician a vanishing species. It is taking much of the fun and challenge out of medicine. It is depersonalizing the doctor-patient relationship. Even worse, it threatens the individuality of patient care.

The day could come when physicians per se will no longer be necessary. In their place will be the ultimate gimmick—a convenience-store computer that takes care of your medical needs and tells your fortune, all for a quarter.

Meanwhile, a reminder. Gimmicks have no judgment or common sense, show no compassion or understanding, and never look at or listen to the patient. A good doctor does.

THE CONSULTATION:
WHO BENEFITS NOW?*

The way we practice medicine is changing. This is understandable considering the growth of medical knowledge, the burgeoning of medical technology, the increasing governmental interventions, the constant threat of litigation, and the growing number of patients we must see with less time to see them in.

While many of the changes undoubtedly benefit the patient, a few seem primarily structured to benefit the doctor. Take, for example, the way we request and give in-hospital consultations.

I remember when the purpose of a consultation was to gain new information or a different perspective. In that light, physicians selected their consultants carefully. The entire process was formal and professional. Doctors communicated with each other directly; they used no go-betweens. The referring physician first obtained permission for consultation from the patient or the family. He then introduced the consultant at the bedside. After the consultant examined the patient, the two

---

*Reprinted by permission from the *Southern Medical Journal* 1985; 78:1145-46.

physicians retired to discuss the case in depth. Together they returned to explain their findings and recommendations to the patient and family. The consultant's official report usually offered pertinent references from the medical literature. If the referring physician disagreed, he often countered with references of his own. This exchange of opinions broadened the diagnostic and therapeutic options. It also contributed to the continuing education of both physicians. The consultant never wrote orders or assumed responsibility for the patient unless the referring physician asked him to and the patient or family approved. Through it all, the referring physician remained firmly in command.

Nowadays, calling in a consultant all too frequently is a way for physicians to save time and thought, protect themselves against malpractice suits, or repay colleagues for previous favors. Consequently, the procedure has lost the planning, formality, and professionalism it once had. Communication between physicians is indirect and impersonal, seldom face to face. "Have Dr. Jones see the patient" or "Surgery consult, stat!" is the message a nurse or ward clerk relays to the consultant. The patient's first inkling of a consultation may be when a stranger enters his room and announces: "I'm Dr. Wizard. I'm an expert on the gizzard." Commonly, the consultant's only link with the referring physician is a scribbled note devoid of medical references. His word becomes gospel, stifling intellectual discourse. He and other consultants take over the patient's care, each concentrating on a part but disregarding the whole. Meanwhile, the referring physician acts as an observer or a triage agent. Everyone—and no one—is in charge.

"So what?" you ask. So I ask, who benefits from this new form of consultation—the patient or the doctor? . . . or neither?

MUTTON'S LAW*

When an enterprising reporter asked Willie Sutton, the notorious bank robber, why he always robbed banks, he reputedly replied, "Because that's where the money is." Willie's logic spurred Dock to coin the term "Sutton's Law" as a reminder for physicians to go where the *diagnosis* is.[1]

Although many patients benefit from Sutton's Law, some profit from a different approach—careful, continued observation. John Milton gave us a way to remember this when he wrote what I call "Milton's Law": "They also serve who only stand and wait."[2]

Thus Sutton's Law encourages specific, well-directed action, while Milton's Law pleads for disciplined, thoughtful inaction. Proper blending of the two is the art of medicine: knowing what to do and when to do it. That's "Mutton's Law."

---

*Reprinted by permission from the *American Heart Journal* 1978; 96:273.

[1]Dock W: Quoted in *Where the Money Was: The Memoirs of a Bank Robber.* Willie Sutton with Edward Linn. New York, Viking Press, 1976, pp. 119-21.

[2]John Milton: On His Blindness. London, 1652.

DIAGNOSTIC
AND THERAPEUTIC TENESMUS*

A serious malady undermines our profession. I call it diagnostic and therapeutic tenesmus. It typically strikes house officers and young practitioners, but even experienced physicians are afflicted. The victims have an uncontrollable urge to diagnose and treat. Without proper attention to the clinical picture, they order a myriad of tests and prescribe a multitude of drugs, hoping to detect and alleviate every possible ill. Their approach is haphazard, time-consuming, unduly expensive, and sometimes dangerous.

What causes this sickness?

Consider today's interns and residents. They enter medical school inquisitive and highly motivated, only to get trapped in a milieu that stifles individuality and discourages intellectual honesty. They also get few chances to see the course of untreated disease; get taught to rely more on the laboratory than on their five senses and their minds; and get little exposure to clinicians who use tests to verify, not to formulate,

---

*Reprinted by permission from the *Southern Medical Journal* 1978; 71:617-18.

impressions. So they leave medical school shackled to routine, with curiosity blunted, and afraid to say "I don't know." No wonder they get tenesmus.

In the older sufferers, attitude is at fault, not training. "With the malpractice crisis, I can't afford to miss anything," they say, or "My patients want it." What patients really want are confident doctors. And doctors who "can't afford to miss anything" do, in fact, miss two things—self-confidence and the joy they once knew making bedside diagnoses.

How do we cure diagnostic and therapeutic tenesmus? By knowing the pathophysiology and natural history of disease. By recognizing that such knowledge demands continuous hard work. By realizing that good patient rapport is the best protection against lawsuits. And by understanding that the debilitating fear of being wrong, not the honest mistake, is our real sin.

"Blessed is the physician who takes a good history, looks keenly at his patient and thinks a bit."[1]

---

[1]Alvarez WC: Quoted in *Walter C. Alvarez: American Man of Medicine.* Scott DH (ed). New York, Van Nostrand Reinhold Co., 1976, p. 8.

MD*

Who shall decide when doctors disagree?
—ALEXANDER POPE, 1732

"MD"—We physicians repeatedly write it, read it, say it, and hear it, but never seem to think about it.

Recently, when I really thought about the letters *MD*, I realized they could have different meanings for different people. A grateful patient, for example, might think of MD as Miracle Doer; a dissatisfied one, as Medical Dummy; a frightened child, as Monstrous Demon. The list of possibilities is endless: Mad Dictator, Millionaire Doctor, Moses Disguised . . .

But for me, MD has a special meaning: *Making Decisions.* Indeed, making medical decisions is what we physicians are licensed and obligated to do. Yet too often we decide not to decide. We shun this basic responsibility and delegate it to a committee of colleagues, to the patient, or to the patient's family.

Making correct decisions in medicine requires

---

*Reprinted by permission from the *Southern Medical Journal* 1978; 71:887.

continually updated scientific knowledge and a skillfully selected data base. But it takes candor and courage, too. Wear MD legitimately. *Make Decisions!*

BUZZWORDS AND BUZZ PROCEDURES*

Can you name ten buzzwords or phrases that we health-care providers say, see, or hear daily? If you're paying attention, you've already seen one that I would name—health-care providers.

My other nominations would be: (2) meaningful dialogue, (3) viable alternatives, (4) risk-benefit ratio, (5) cost-effective, (6) state-of-the-art, and the ever-popular (7) prioritize, (8) optimize, and (9) finalize. The tenth— *noninvasive*— prompts this commentary.

Noninvasive—what does it mean? I posed that question to several colleagues, house officers, and medical students, asking them to classify specific procedures as invasive or noninvasive. As I expected, they all viewed electrocardiography and ultrasonography as noninvasive and all considered cardiac catheterization and carotid arteriography as invasive. But they varied considerably in their classification of bronchoscopy, barium enema, radionuclide studies, and simple venipuncture.

Next I went to the dictionary, which defines *noninvasive* as "not involving penetration (as by surgery

---

*Reprinted by permission from *Houston Medical Journal* 1986; 2:42-43.

or hypodermic needle) of the skin of the intact organism." Conversely, it defines *invasive* as "involving entry into the living body (as by incision or by insertion of an instrument)." The more I reflected on these definitions, the more I agreed with Spodick, who said, "I think the designation 'noninvasive' should mean exactly what it says, that is, that the body is not penetrated in any way."[1]

The fact is, we doctors regularly invade our patients in one way or another, though we don't always perceive it as such. We invade their privacy by the medical histories we take and the physical examinations we do. We puncture their skin to draw blood. We stick catheters into their bladders, put tubes down their throats, place speculums in their vaginas, and insert scopes up their rectums. And most of what we do invades their pocketbooks.

Why, then, is "noninvasiveness" so in vogue? One reason is the ever-increasing array of new, highly touted, and widely available noninvasive procedures. Another is the potential of these procedures to enhance patient care. A third is the specter of litigation.

Doctors are flocking to the noninvasive approach in the belief that it offers greater physical safety for their patients and greater legal safety for themselves. But noninvasive procedures are not always as reliable as their invasive counterparts. And there is some feeling that our new technology is "insufficiently validated, irresponsibly disseminated and uncritically accepted."[2] Noninvasive procedures, therefore, can lead the unwary

---

[1]Spodick DH: When "noninvasive" means "invasive." *Annals Intern Med* 92:722, 1980.

[2]Diamond GA: Monkey business. *Am J Cardiol* 57:471-75, 1986.

toward blissful misdiagnosis and catastrophic mismanagement. Thus, we have a paradox: noninvasiveness itself can be dangerous.

These remarks have but one purpose—to make us think about the buzzwords we use and the "buzz procedures" we choose. Buzzwords and buzz procedures are effective only to the extent that we know their limitations.

To finalize, we health-care providers should initiate meaningful dialogue on buzzwords and seek viable alternatives to them. In accordance with the state-of-the-art, we should also prioritize our selection of buzz procedures. The risk-benefit ratio of such efforts would be cost-effective and would optimize patient care.

THE REAL QUESTION*

Scene I. A party.

The conversation typically begins like this:

"And what do you do?"

"I'm a physician," I say.

"What kind of doctor are you?"

"A good one, I hope!"

That answer startles many people; they expect to hear the traditional "I'm a surgeon," or pediatrician, or whatever. And, in this setting, the concept of a good doctor is really not important to them.

Scene II. Anyplace, sometime later.

The same people are facing illness, and they ask, "Is so-and-so a good doctor?" or "Can you recommend a good doctor?" Now the concept of a good doctor *is* important to them.

Epilogue.

A good doctor? From my standpoint, the real question is not so much *who,* but *what,* is a good doctor. I believe a good doctor blends compassion with candor, book

---

*Reprinted by permission from *Forum on Medicine* 1979; 2:579.

sense with common sense. He strives diligently to maintain perspective, focusing on the patient, not the disease. He always finds time to listen to those seeking his help; perceives more than just their words; and talks with, not to, them in an easily understood way. He thinks for himself and makes his own decisions. He relies chiefly on his mind and five senses for diagnoses; knows the indications for and limitations of laboratory procedures; and uses tests and consultants to verify, not formulate, his clinical impressions. He respects and appreciates nurses, technicians, and other members of the health-care team. And, cognizant of his own fallibility, he is never afraid to say, "I don't know."

When the Bell Doesn't Ring*

A friend called me long-distance recently to discuss a diagnostic problem. "I'm stumped," he said, "and I need your help. I've got this forty-three-year-old woman with migratory thrombophlebitis limited to her arms. Initially, I thought she had a painful epitrochlear node, but on resection the 'node' turned out to be a large thrombosed vein. After that, similar nodules developed in the opposite arm. I've done everything to find cancer or a collagen disease. But all the tests are negative, and she doesn't respond to anticoagulant or steroid therapy. In fact, one of the lesions came on while she was receiving steroids."

"Let me think about this," I replied.

As I reflected on our conversation, something didn't ring true. So I phoned him for more details. In response to my specific questions, he reported that the patient was a widow who worked as a nurse's aide in the local hospital. She seemed emotionally stable and gave no history of substance abuse. Her lesions were confined not just to her arms, but to her antecubital spaces. They

---

*Reprinted by permission from *Houston Medical Journal* 1987; 3:38-39.

would appear abruptly as small, rounded masses; become red, warm, minimally raised, and tender; grow rapidly to the size of a quarter; and resolve slowly, leaving a sclerotic, ropy base. During a month of observation, five lesions occurred on the right arm and one on the left, with a maximum of two at any given time. The patient is right-handed.

In light of this additional information, three things stood out: the doctor was baffled; the lesions were bizarre; and the patient was a female with a medically related job and a peculiar illness. Each of these circumstances alone should suggest factitious disease;[1] together, they make the diagnosis almost certain. Nevertheless, I did consider the nodular form of spontaneous thrombophlebitis, also known as primary recurrent idiopathic thrombophlebitis or thrombophlebitis migrans. This disorder, however, primarily involves small and medium-sized veins, predominantly affects men, and characteristically manifests itself on the legs.[2] I also considered erythema nodosum,[3] subcutaneous fat necrosis,[4] autoerythrocyte

---

[1]Reich P, Gottfried LA: Factitious disorders in a teaching hospital. *Ann Intern Med* 99:240-47, 1983.

Price WA, Giannini AJ: Factitious anemia: Case reports and literature review. *Psychiatr Forum* Winter 1985–1986, pp. 60-64.

Aduan RP, Fauci AS, Dale DC, et al.: Factitious fever and self-induced infection. A report of 32 cases and review of the literature. *Ann Intern Med* 90:230-42, 1979.

[2]Montgomery H, O'Leary PA, Barker NW: Nodular vascular diseases of the legs. Erythema induratum and allied conditions. *JAMA* 128:335-41, 1945.

Allen EV, Barker NW, Hines EA Jr: *Peripheral Vascular Diseases,* 2d ed. Philadelphia, W. B. Saunders Company, 1955, pp. 499-500.

[3]Tierney LM Jr, Schwartz RA: Erythema nodosum. *Am Fam Physician*

sensitization syndrome,[5] Behcet's disease,[6] and a primary infectious process.[7] Because the first biopsy might not have been adequate or representative of the succeeding lesions, I advised biopsy of a fresh nodule and requested that all tissue sections be sent to me.

Three weeks later, I received slide preparations from the original biopsy and from a subsequent biopsy. I presented them as unknowns to our chief pathologist, who indicated that both biopsies showed conspicuously large veins with intensely inflamed, slightly thickened walls surrounding newly formed, non-occluding thrombi. The adjacent fat and overlying skin were normal, and no foreign material or organisms were evident. He wondered whether the patient was a drug addict, and on learning the clinical findings, immediately favored self-induced injury. The patient's doctor, meanwhile, had reached the same conclusion.

Difficulty in this case arose because my friend did what all of us do from time to time—focused on a part and lost sight of the whole. He zeroed in on thrombophlebitis, and in searching for its cause, didn't

---

30:227-32, 1984.

Weinstein L: Erythema nodosum. *Disease-of-the-Month,* June 1984, pp. 1-30.

[4]Hughes PSH, Apisarnthanarax P, Mullins JF: Subcutaneous fat necrosis associated with pancreatic disease. *Arch Dermatol* 111:506-10, 1975.

[5]Ratnoff OD, Agle DP: Psychogenic purpura: A re-evaluation of the syndrome of autoerythrocyte sensitization. *Medicine* 47:475-500, 1968.

[6]O'Duffy JD, Carney JA, Deodhar S: Behcet's disease. Report of 10 cases, 3 with new manifestations. *Ann Intern Med* 75:561-70, 1971.

[7]Moore P, Willkens RF: The subcutaneous nodule: Its significance in the diagnosis of rheumatic disease. *Sem Arthritis Rheumatol* 7:63-79, 1977.

see the link between his own puzzlement, the location of the lesions, and the patient's sex and occupation.

When the right diagnostic bell doesn't ring, you may be in the wrong belfry.

CANCER SOMEWHERE*

The opportunities for physicians to make correct diagnoses have increased progressively with advances in medical knowledge, improved teaching facilities and curricula, more rapid dissemination of scientific information, and the availability of many new diagnostic technics of great specificity. While one cannot gainsay the salutary effects of these changes, an incorrect diagnosis is not a rare event. It seems plausible, however, that the physician might be fallible less often if he appreciated the common sources of diagnostic error.

Gruver and Freis found that preventable mistakes in diagnosis resulted primarily from failure to (a) account for abnormal symptoms, signs, or laboratory reports that did not fit with the clinical impression; (b) obtain routine screening tests or perform other indicated procedures; (c) realize that roentgen studies may not disclose pathologic changes; (d) recognize new illnesses developing in the presence of a previously diagnosed chronic disease; and (e) review periodically the records of patients with prolonged illnesses and/or repeat the

---

*Reprinted by permission from *Medical Times* 1965; 93:735-38.

physical examination.[1] They emphasized that malignant tumors frequently were mistaken for other diseases but did not mention the problem of other diseases masquerading as cancer. In this regard, we have been interested in those cases in which the physician may be prompted to remark, "This patient probably has a cancer somewhere." It has been our experience that such a clinical impression is more often wrong than right. Furthermore, we maintain that the phrase "cancer somewhere" is arbitrary, uninformative, and misleading and that it indicates lack of critical thought or an inability to do the simple things properly. To support this contention we will present several examples of the "cancer somewhere" syndrome, emphasizing in each case the lessons to be learned.

Report of Cases

Case 1

A middle-aged woman was subjected to total thyroidectomy for benign goiter. Four months later ascites developed rapidly. On physical examination the patient was wasted and had "that malignancy look." Her abdomen was tightly distended with fluid. The initial clinical impression was "ascites secondary to metastatic tumor, site of origin unknown." Roentgen examination of the chest and gastrointestinal tract showed no abnormality. The results of liver function tests and biopsy were normal. The serum protein bound iodine was 1.4μg. per 100 ml. The peritoneal fluid contained four gm of protein per 100 ml but no cells. Thyroid replacement therapy was begun, but the patient died

---

[1]Gruver RH, Freis ED: A study of diagnostic errors. *Ann Intern Med* 47:108-20, 1957.

twenty days later. Careful necropsy disclosed a large amount of ascitic fluid for which no cause could be found. Presumably, the ascites was a manifestation of the hypothyroidism.[2]

Comment

This case illustrates the fallacy of basing one's clinical impression of cancer solely on the presence of ascites and/or "that cancer look." Indeed, "cancer somewhere" all too often is diagnosed in an attempt to explain away the presence of cachexia even though many other illnesses may lead to emaciation.

Case 2

An old man was admitted to the hospital five times in five months because of tense ascites of unknown cause. Thorough medical history and physical examination revealed no evidence of disease other than ascites. Tests of liver function (Bromsulphalein® retention, thymol turbidity, cephalin cholesterol flocculation, prothrombin time and serum albumin, globulin, glutamic oxaloacetic transaminase, alkaline phosphatase, and bilirubin) and roentgenograms of the entire alimentary tract disclosed no abnormality. The ascitic fluid was a transudate in which no malignant cells were identified. Nevertheless, carcinomatosis with peritoneal seeding was thought to be the cause of the ascites. The patient finally consented to exploratory celiotomy which showed massive ascites and postnecrotic cirrhosis without evidence of malignancy.

---

[2]Kocen RS, Atkinson M: Ascites in hypothyroidism. *Lancet* 1:527-30, 1963.

Comment

Ascites rarely is the sole presenting manifestation of carcinomatosis, except in some women with ovarian malignancy. As a matter of fact, if a large amount of free intra-abdominal fluid is the only finding suggesting cancer, another cause for that fluid should be sought. Indeed, when ascites is the patient's outstanding clinical feature, hepatic cirrhosis is the most common underlying disorder.[3] Also, it is well documented that even in patients with advanced hepatic disease, results of liver function tests may be normal.[4]

Case 3

A forty-seven-year-old white woman had had a right nephrectomy at age thirty-five for a hypernephroma. At the age of forty-four, she was treated with radium and x-irradiation for carcinoma of the cervix. Shortly before she came under our care, the patient lost thirty pounds in two months. Her gynecologist admitted her to the hospital where his examination disclosed an enlarged liver, signs of weight loss, and anemia. He diagnosed advanced cancer and referred the patient for chemotherapy.

A more detailed medical history revealed heat intolerance, emotional lability, increased sweating, nervousness, sleeplessness, and palpitation during the preceding year. The patient's appetite had been good but not excessive. She did not fatigue easily and had no

---

[3]Berner C, Fred HL, Riggs S, and David JS: Diagnostic probabilities in patients with conspicuous ascites. *Arch Intern Med* 113:687-90, 1964.

[4]Gross JB, Dockerty MB: Hepatic enlargement with normal excretion of sulfobromophthalein: Some diagnostic experiences with needle biopsy of the liver. *Proc Mayo Clin* 37:83-94, 1962.

abdominal discomfort. Physical examination disclosed a regular pulse at a rate of 120 beats per minute and weight of 107 pounds. The patient moved about constantly and had a slight stare, warm skin, and a fine tremor of her hands. Her thyroid gland was diffusely enlarged to twice normal size. A smooth, nontender hepatic edge was palpable two cm below the right costal margin. Pelvic examination disclosed no abnormality. A diagnosis of thyrotoxicosis was made and was confirmed by a twenty-four-hour I^{131} uptake of 75 percent. After treatment with radioactive iodine, the patient gained weight. For two years now, she has been asymptomatic and free of evident disease.

Comment

This case exemplifies the pitfall of a prejudiced viewpoint,[5] that is, allowing the knowledge of a previously confirmed diagnosis of malignant disease to bias the physician's evaluation of the patient's current illness. It also points out that the surest way to "cure" cancer is to change the diagnosis.

Case 4

An old man's sole complaint was progressive weakness of three months' duration. On physical examination pallor was the only abnormality. The hematocrit value was 22 ml/100 ml and the total leukocyte count was 6,000 per cu mm. On the assumption that anemia of this magnitude in an elderly patient most likely resulted from a bleeding intestinal tumor, extensive diagnostic studies were undertaken. Results of stool guaiac tests, roentgenograms of the gastrointestinal tract,

---

[5]Gruver, Freis: Study of diagnostic errors.

and sigmoidoscopy were normal. Pernicious anemia was believed the next most likely diagnosis, but examination of the gastric juice disclosed the presence of free acid. At this point serious attention was directed for the first time to the patient's peripheral blood film. The erythrocytes were normocytic and normochromic, not microcytic and hypochromic as one would expect with chronic intestinal bleeding. Neither were they macrocytic as one ordinarily finds in patients with pernicious anemia. More important still, there were immature leukocytes diagnostic of acute monomyeloblastic leukemia.

Comment

Because anemia frequently accompanies malignancy, its presence in middle-aged or elderly patients too often is considered the result of "cancer until proven otherwise." This assumption may precipitate costly and debilitating examinations of the alimentary and urinary tracts when a more carefully performed physical examination and simple but critically conducted hematologic studies would establish the proper diagnosis. In this particular case the patient did have a "cancer somewhere," but its specific identification was delayed unnecessarily. Failure to examine critically the peripheral blood film of an anemic patient is a common but inexcusable error.

Case 5

An elderly woman complained of nausea, vomiting, weight loss, and weakness. She appeared pale and wasted and had fever, hepatomegaly, and minimal icterus. The initial clinical impression was "metastatic carcinoma, site of origin unknown." Numerous diagnostic procedures were scheduled. Before these were carried out, however, more discerning physical examination revealed a smooth tongue and palpable spleen. Pernicious anemia was suspected and confirmed.

Comment

Some "C A" is "P A."

Conclusions

We recognize that there are patients with symptomatic malignancy in whom the diagnosis cannot be proved without prolonged observation and/or exhaustive study. In many others, however, a thorough medical history and careful physical examination correlated with the results of routine blood count, urinalysis, stool guaiac test, roentgenogram of the chest, and a knowledge of the manifestations and natural histories of common neoplastic diseases will enable the physician to decide on the likelihood of cancer as well as its probable type, site of origin, and extent of spread. He then is able to select those few appropriate additional studies that can lead him to a precise diagnosis. Such an approach is reliable, simple, inexpensive, and direct. Conscientiously pursued, it renders needless or absurd the loosely applied, often erroneous, and sometimes dangerous diagnosis of "cancer somewhere."

— Herbert L. Fred, M.D.

—John M. Eiband, M.D.

—Montague Lane, M.D.

From the Department of Internal Medicine, Baylor University College of Medicine, Houston, Texas

Washing Our Hands of the Matter*

A century and a half ago, Semmelweis concluded that students performing autopsies on victims of puerperal fever were carrying the infection to healthy mothers in the obstetrical ward.[1] He believed, in turn, that washing one's hands with soap and water before examining women in labor would be lifesaving. History proved him right.

Subsequent investigators have shown that contaminated hands can transmit organisms capable of causing respiratory, urinary, cutaneous, enteric, or surgical wound infections.[2] Thus, handwashing today is

---

*Reprinted by permission from *Houston Medical Journal* 1987; 3:75-76.

[1]*Encyclopaedia Britannica,* vol. 20, Chicago, William Benton, 1965, p. 318.

[2]Goodman RA: Nosocomial hepatitis A. *Ann Intern Med* 103:452-54, 1985.

Steere AC, Mallison GF: Handwashing practices for the prevention of nosocomial infections. *Ann Intern Med* 83:683-90, 1975.

Gwaltney JM Jr, Moskalski PB, Hendley JO: Hand-to-hand transmission of rhinovirus colds. *Ann Intern Med* 88:463-67, 1978.

an integral part of preventing and controlling contagion.[3] And though numerous disinfectants are available, plain soap and running water will remove the majority of transiently acquired organisms.[4]

During my medical training in the early 1950s, I was taught to wash my hands after examining every patient, whether the patient was well or sick, clean or dirty. I still adhere to that policy, but I find few colleagues who do. Indeed, studies confirm that hospital personnel are lax in their handwashing techniques,[5] physicians being among the worst offenders.[6]

---

[3]Steere, Mallison: Handwashing practices.

Sprunt K, Redman W, Leidy G: Antibacterial effectiveness of routine hand washing. *Pediatrics* 52:264-71, 1973.

Favero MS, Maynard JE, Leger RT: Prevention and control of infections in specialized areas—Viral hepatitis. *Crit Care Q* 3:43-55, 1980.

Williams WW: Guideline for infection control in hospital personnel. *Infect Control* 4:329-49, 1983.

Jeffries D: ABC of AIDS: Control of infection policies. *Br Med J* 295:33-35, 1987.

[4]Steere, Mallison: Handwashing practices.

Center for Disease Control: *National Nosocomial Infections Study Quarterly Report.* Third and Fourth Quarters 1973, issued March 1975, pp. 19-28.

[5]Steere, Mallison: Handwashing practices.

Center for Disease Control: *National Nosocomial Infections.*

Preston GA, Larson EL, Stamm WE: The effect of private isolation rooms on patient care practices, colonization and infection in an intensive care unit. *Am J Med* 70:641-45, 1981.

Goodman RA, Carder CC, Allen JR, et al.: Nosocomial hepatitis A transmission by an adult patient with diarrhea. *Am J Med* 73:220-26, 1982.

Fox MK, Langner SB, Wells RW: How good are hand washing practices? *Am J Nursing* 74:1676-78, 1974.

Robertson WO: Hand washing in hospitals (*Letter*). *N Engl J Med* 305:963, 1981.

[6]Albert RK, Condie F: Hand-washing patterns in medical intensive-care units. *N Engl J Med* 304:1465-66, 1981.

The general public is also guilty of poor handwashing habits. The next time you're in a locker room or restroom, note that many people *don't* wash their hands after using the toilet. Some of these individuals carry disease, which they can disseminate in various ways, especially by preparing or serving food. But they aren't likely to wash their hands *when* they should until they learn *why* they should. In that light, we in the medical profession can help by spreading the word—and then practicing what we preach.

So: instead of "washing our hands of the matter," let's all wash our hands of the "matter."

MAGNETIC RESONANCE IMAGING: A PATIENT'S ENDORSEMENT*

If a technique enables doctors to peer inside the human body noninvasively, it attracts attention. If that technique is also exceptionally sensitive, uses no ionizing radiation, and has no proven side effects, it deserves attention. And if that technique has the added potential of precisely identifying, localizing, and monitoring the physiologic, metabolic, and pathologic features of tissues in vivo,[1] it commands attention. Such a technique is Magnetic Resonance Imaging (MRI). In this essay, I endorse MRI—not as a basic scientist, medical-imaging specialist, or clinician, but as a physician-patient who benefited greatly from this ingenious technologic advance.

Six months ago, I was crossing a busy downtown intersection, about to finish my daily run, when a

---

*Reprinted by permission from *Houston Medical Journal* 1987; 3:115-17.

[1]Anderson M: Nuclear magnetic resonance imaging and neurology. *Br Med J* 284:1359-60, 1982.

motorist coming from my left ran a red light and hit me. The collision bent the car's front bumper and right front fender, and my head shattered the windshield.
I remember the moment of impact; it was painless. The next thing I knew I was lying on the pavement looking skyward, noting the clouds rolling round and around. Seconds later my head, left shoulder, right rib cage, and left foot began to hurt.

No broken bones were evident, despite an extensive roentgenographic search. Computed tomographic (CT) scan of my head disclosed normal-sized ventricles and no mass effect, midline shift, or hemorrhage. The study, however, didn't include the two uppermost slices because I couldn't cooperate fully. My diagnosis at admission was concussion with widespread soft tissue injuries.

During the next few days, I complained bitterly of unremitting and progressively severe bifrontal headache and persistent pain in my shoulder, rib cage, and foot. Additionally, my sense of taste and smell vanished, and I refused all food and liquids. My doctors suspected a subdural hematoma and ordered another CT scan of my head (without contrast) seven days after the initial one. This time the scan included the top two slices. It demonstrated a nondisplaced paramedian fracture in the left frontal region but no other abnormality. Later that day, MRI of my brain unveiled a small subdural hematoma beneath the fracture, minimal compression of the contiguous cerebral cortex, and multiple hemorrhages in both temporal and frontal lobes, especially on the left.

Armed with this new information, my doctors gave me steroids intravenously. My excruciating headache disappeared within twenty-four hours and has not recurred. I went home after eleven days.

Subsequent x-ray examinations uncovered fractures in my left foot, left scapula, and right rib cage. MRI done fifty-eight days after the original study showed resolution of the subdural hematoma and clearing of all hemorrhages except for a small amount in the tip of the left frontal lobe. My sense of taste returned rapidly, but my sense of smell remains impaired.

This story illustrates what every seasoned physician knows: normal test results do not necessarily exclude disease at the site of persistent, localized pain— particularly when the pain is in an area recently traumatized. Conventional roentgenograms of my left shoulder, for example, were repeatedly normal. But the continuing pain in my shoulder prompted the radiologist to obtain an uncommon view that displayed a through-and-through crack of the acromion.

Similarly, though my worsening headache suggested a subdural hematoma, the follow-up CT scan failed to delineate any intracranial abnormality. The radiologist, therefore, recommended MRI. I'm thankful he did, because the findings from MRI effected an abrupt turnabout in my care, resulting in immediate clinical improvement and more enlightened long-term management. Those findings not only explained my headache and my absent sense of smell, but also set forth reasons why I shouldn't drive a car or resume vigorous exercise until the intracranial complications had largely resolved. And in cases like mine, MRI is the safest, most accurate way to document such resolution.

For studying the central nervous system, MRI has certain advantages over CT scanning.[2] It is distinctly more sensitive in detecting many types of intracranial lesions;[3] generates transverse, saggital, and coronal images as required;[4] and provokes no signal from the skull, which allows the surface of the adjacent brain to be seen clearly.[5] It also provides a higher degree of contrast between gray and white matter.[6]

MRI has drawbacks, too. It is contraindicated in patients unable to lie motionless or who have intracranial aneurysm clips, cardiac pacemakers, or monitoring equipment that incorporates ferromagnetic substances. Moreover, patients with claustrophobia will find this examination intolerable. To me, it felt like being buried alive. My head barely fit into a rigid "cage," and my body barely fit into a long, dark tube. The noise accompanying the procedure—mimicking both machine gun and slow rifle fire—was so loud that I wore ear plugs. And MRI is expensive.

---

[2]Steiner RE: Nuclear magnetic resonance imaging. *Br Med J* 294:1570-72, 1987.

[3]Lye RH, Ramsden RT, Stack JP, Gillespie JE: Trigeminal nerve tumor: Comparison of CT and MRI. Case Report. *J Neurosurg* 67:124-27, 1987.

[4]Anderson: Nuclear magnetic resonance imaging.

[5]Ibid.

[6]Steiner: Nuclear magnetic resonance imaging.

As I reflect on my accident, I think about the innumerable patients in years past in whom the diagnosis of "concussion" was as finite as technology permitted. Some of them surely had intracranial complications comparable to mine. But those patients didn't have access to MRI. Fortunately, I did.

Don't Just Do Something—
Stand There*

The message from my wife was clear: "There's something wrong with Greg's neck. Come home now."

As usual, Greg—our six-year-old—was waiting for me at the back door. But this time, he didn't jump up for his hug. He couldn't. He was holding his head down and to the left. If he tried to move it or I tried to touch it, he would cry out in pain.

In retrospect, Greg had been irritable and less active for a few weeks, and his neck had seemed a little stiff. The acute pain, however, was new. His gait, too, was different— shuffling and unsteady.

Fearing the worst, I took Greg directly to his doctor. After quizzing me and examining Greg, the doctor listed as possibilities degenerative disease of the spinal cord, ruptured cervical disk, cervical arthritis, and cancer of the spine. He believed that the specific cause had to be identified and treated promptly. Otherwise, incapacitating, irreversible neurologic complications

---

*Reprinted by permission from the *Southern Medical Journal* 1988; 81:1162-63.

might ensue. He therefore urged immediate neurosurgical consultation.

An hour later I was talking by phone with a neurosurgeon. On hearing the story, he recommended sedation, immobilization, pain medication, and a myelogram. He thought that an operation on Greg's neck might become necessary.

The seriousness of the matter persuaded me to take Greg to the university medical center 100 miles away. There I could receive additional opinions, and if surgical intervention did prove necessary, Greg would have a team of specialists to care for him—advantages not available locally.

When we arrived at the university outpatient clinic, a student and the chief surgical resident met us. They befriended Greg while I filled out an extensive form detailing his medical history. Next, they gave him an impressively thorough physical examination. The chief resident then called in the professor of neurology/neurosurgery, Dr. Patricia Luttgen.

She assessed the situation and examined Greg. "Dr. Fred," she said, "I suggest that you leave Greg with us for a few days. I promise to watch him carefully. We may do a myelogram tomorrow, but we won't do anything else without your knowledge and approval. I'll keep you apprised of Greg's progress and call you when I've reached a conclusion."

Dr. Luttgen's call brought good news—news that was startling and somewhat embarrassing. Greg was fine! His neck and gait were normal. In fact, he had run tirelessly and painlessly in a field playing ball with Dr. Luttgen. He also seemed pleased by all of the affection that the students and house officers had shown him. And he had undergone no testing aside from a routine blood count and urinalysis. No myelogram, no operation.

When my wife and I came to pick up our youngster, Dr. Luttgen told us that his problem was loneliness. Holding his neck in a strange position and intermittently crying out in pain was his way of gaining the attention and love that he wasn't getting.

Everything made sense, especially when I saw the improvement in Greg's appearance and attitude. Tincture of time and love had done wonders for him. I couldn't help but think what might have happened had I not decided to seek help from the College of Veterinary Medicine at Texas A & M University. For if you haven't guessed, Greg is our Doberman pinscher.

Baron von Gregory is nine years old now. Since his hospitalization he occasionally holds his neck down, whines, and begins to wobble. But if we give him an extra hug, tell him how much we love him, or give him a bone, those manifestations vanish.

The way the veterinarians at Texas A & M University handled Greg is the way we physicians ought to handle our patients—take a good history, do a pertinent physical examination, and then think a bit. That's always safer, and cheaper, than jumping immediately to a lot of tests. In that light, Greg's total bill for five days in the hospital was an incredible $107. And that included the professional fees!

This story exemplifies the medical value of what I call "Milton's Law"[1]: "They also serve who only stand and wait."[2] Indeed, by standing and waiting, Dr. Luttgen and her associates served Greg well—they gave him a new "leash" on life.

---

[1]Fred HL: Mutton's law. *Am Heart J* 96:273, 1978.

[2]John Milton: On his blindness. London, 1652.

DIAGNOSTIC PLEASURES REVISITED: PART I*

Medicine has changed. We doctors formerly used our minds and five senses to make diagnoses. Now we use machines. We find it more convenient and believe it is legally safer to order tests before we put our thoughts in order. Too often we check a blood gas rather than examine the lungs; obtain an echocardiogram instead of listening carefully to the heart; and rely on consultants to make decisions for us. The coveted patient-doctor relationship has taken a back seat to the lawyer-patient bond. No wonder medicine has lost its fun—at least for me.

As I reflect on the time when medicine *was* fun, I recall many unusual and challenging patients. Most of them had disorders best appreciated by photographs or by detailed descriptions of their case histories. A few, however, had illnesses that the informed physician can diagnose or strongly suspect from the following clues.

• A Ute Indian underwent drainage of a perirectal abscess. During the next few months, he experienced asymptomatic, odorless destruction of his entire

*Reprinted by permission from *Houston Medicine* 1988; 4:87-88.

perineum and scrotum. The process eventually lay bare his testes and ischial bones. Repeated biopsies and cultures of the affected tissues shed no light on the cause, and despite administration of multiple antibiotics, he died.

• A middle-aged white woman developed a generalized purplish hue and lanugo-type facial hair. Nine months later, at the time of her death, she had turned black.

• An elderly woman had a knee that was warm—almost hot—to the touch but painless and normal in appearance. These findings did not change during three years of follow-up.

• A young woman complained of increasing difficulty reading fine print. While testing her strength, I had her squeeze my hand. It took her five seconds to let go.

• Two vagrants hopped a freight train in Reno, Nevada—drunk, but otherwise O.K. On arriving in Salt Lake City the next day, one was dead and the other was blind.

Finally, these patients:

• A man who had brown sweat and blue eardrums;

• A teenager who had a pulsating varicocele;

• A boxer who had intense scleral icterus but whose serum bilirubin concentration was normal;

• A boy who could smile but couldn't whistle;

• And a woman who could whistle but couldn't smile.

In my next column, I will furnish the diagnosis and cite one or more reference articles for each disorder listed. I will also name any respondents who, in the interim, correctly account for the abnormalities described. For them, the prize will be the satisfaction of having met the challenge *without* resorting to the laboratory.

Diagnostic Pleasures Revisited: Concluded*

In the preceding issue (*Houston Medicine* 1988; 4:87-88), I described some of my unusual and challenging patients from years past. The descriptions, however, included only the salient clinical features of each case. Now, as promised, I will furnish the diagnoses and cite pertinent reference articles.

CASE: After undergoing drainage of a perirectal abscess, a Ute Indian experienced progressive destruction of his entire perineum. Repeated biopsies and cultures of the affected tissues gave no diagnosis, and despite therapy with multiple antibiotics, the patient died.

Comment: Careful autopsy examination uncovered no explanation for this man's illness. So, to the chagrin of everyone involved, including the chairmen of Medicine, Surgery, and Pathology at the medical school, the case ended without an answer.

Several months later, while on duty one night, I saw a medical journal lying open at the nurses' station. Amazingly, it showed a picture of a man whose ulcerated

---

*Reprinted by permission from *Houston Medicine* 1988; 4:127-30.

perineum appeared strikingly similar to the perineum of my patient. The diagnosis in that case was cutaneous amebiasis.

I immediately called the staff pathologist who had interpreted the numerous biopsies and had done the autopsy on my patient. He came back to the hospital and at midnight looked for amebic trophozoites in the slides previously obtained. He found them in nearly every section reviewed.

REFERENCES

Song YS. Cutaneous amebiasis: Report of two cases with one autopsy. *Ann Intern Med* 1956; 44:1211-18.
(*Note:* This article led to the diagnosis in my patient's case.)

Davson J, Jones DM, Turner L. Diagnosis of Meleney's synergistic gangrene. *Br J Surg* 1988; 75:267-71.
(*Note:* This review emphasizes that Meleney's postoperative progressive synergistic gangrene is indistinguishable clinically from cutaneous amebiasis. It also provides strong evidence that many cases previously called Meleney's gangrene were, in fact, amebic gangrene. Amebic trophozoites are easy to miss in sections stained by hematoxylin and eosin; they are also easily confused with macrophages.)

McConaghey RMS. Amoebiasis of the anus and perineum. With report of a case. *Indian Medical Gazette* 1945; 80:79-81.

CASE: A middle-aged white woman developed a generalized purplish hue with lanugo-type facial hair. By the time of her death nine months later, she had turned black.

Comment: This woman had proven metastatic malignant melanoma with intense deposits of melanin throughout her skin and internal organs. Her lanugo-type facial hair was an early cutaneous marker of internal malignancy.

REFERENCES

Trueblood DV. Malignant melanoma with generalized skin blackening. The white girl who turned black. *Northwest Med* 1947; 46:199-202.

Fitzpatrick TB, Montgomery H, Lerner AB. Pathogenesis of generalized dermal pigmentation secondary to malignant melanoma and melanuria. *J Invest Dermatol* 1954; 22:163-72.

Wadskov S, Bro-Jørgensen A, Søndergaard J. Acquired hypertrichosis lanuginosa: A skin marker of internal malignancy. *Arch Dermatol* 1976; 112:1442-44.

CASE: An elderly white woman had a knee warm to the touch but painless and normal in appearance over a three-year span.

Comment: A roentgenogram disclosed Paget's disease of the knee. Paget's disease can cause increased regional blood flow up to twenty times normal, resulting in warm limbs and sometimes redness of the skin in the involved areas. Pain is often absent, and affected joints need not be enlarged or deformed.

REFERENCES

Rhodes BA, Greyson ND, Hamilton CR Jr, et al. Absence of anatomic arteriovenous shunts in Paget's disease of bone. *N Engl J Med* 1972; 287:686-89.

Franck WA, Bress NM, Singer FR, Krane SM. Rheumatic manifestations of Paget's disease of bone. *Am J Med* 1974; 56:592-603.

CASE: A young woman complained of difficulty reading fine print. On physical examination, she had trouble relaxing her grip.

Comment: She had myotonic dystrophy, the cardinal feature of which is persistence of muscle contraction after active motion. When these patients shake your hand, they cannot let go quickly. Additionally, they frequently have a characteristic type of cataract that may affect their vision.

REFERENCES

Perkoff GT, Tyler FH. The differential diagnosis of progressive muscular dystrophy. *Med Clin North Am* 1953; 37:545-63.

Burian HM, Burns CA. Ocular changes in myotonic dystrophy. *Am J Ophthalmol* 1967; 63:22-34.

CASE: Two vagrants became drunk, and by the next day, one had died and the other had become blind.

Comment: This is a classic story of methyl alcohol poisoning. The survivor admitted drinking illicit whiskey the day before, but couldn't remember what happened after that. On examination, he was acidotic, with reddened optic discs and retinal edema.

REFERENCE

Bennett IL Jr, Cary FH, Mitchell GL Jr, Cooper MN. Acute methyl alcohol poisoning: A review based on experiences in an outbreak of 323 cases. *Medicine* 1953; 32:431-63.

CASE: A man had brown sweat and blue eardrums.

Comment: This man also passed black urine. Such a technicolored combination of findings is typical of alcaptonuria with ochronosis.

REFERENCE

O'Brien WM, La Du BN, Bunim JJ. Biochemical, pathologic and clinical aspects of alcaptonuria, ochronosis and ochronotic arthropathy. Review of world literature (1584–1962). *Am J Med* 1963; 34:813-38.

CASE: A teenager had a pulsating varicocele.

Comment: Pulsatile varicose veins are virtually pathognomonic of tricuspid insufficiency. This teenager had rheumatic heart disease with tricuspid insufficiency. I have seen another youngster with a pulsating varicocele consequent to the tricuspid insufficiency of Ebstein's anomaly.

REFERENCE

Brickner PW, Scudder WT, Weinrib M. Pulsating varicose veins in functional tricuspid insufficiency. Case report and venous pressure tracing. *Circulation* 1962; 25:126-29.

CASE: A boxer had scleral icterus with normal serum bilirubin concentration.

Comment: One week earlier, this man had sustained two black eyes along with bilateral subconjunctival hemorrhage. As such hemorrhage absorbs, it goes through a series of chromatic changes owing to breakdown of blood pigments. About seven or more days after the bleeding episode, the affected sclerae can appear deeply icteric.

REFERENCE

Adler FH. *Gifford's Textbook of Ophthalmology,* 4th edition. Philadelphia: W. B. Saunders Company, 1948, pp. 199-200.

CASE: A boy could smile but couldn't whistle.

Comment: Asymmetrical involvement of the orbicularis oris muscles is an early manifestation of progressive muscular dystrophy of the facioscapulohumeral type. The resultant inability to pucker the lips prohibits whistling and is characteristic of the disorder.

REFERENCE

Perkoff GT, Tyler FH. The differential diagnosis of progressive muscular dystrophy. *Med Clin North Am* 1953; 37:545-63.

CASE: A woman could whistle but couldn't smile.

Comment: This patient had advanced scleroderma. The skin of her face was so tight that she could barely open her mouth. Yet she could muster a faint whistle by placing her tongue against her front teeth and exhaling forcibly.

REFERENCE

Leinwand I, Duryee AW, Richter MN. Scleroderma (Based on a study of over 150 cases). *Ann Intern Med* 1954; 41:1003-40.

EPILOGUE

Though nobody submitted the right diagnoses for all of these patients, one came close. Dr. Ken Sack, professor of medicine, the University of California at San Francisco, identified every disorder except the cutaneous amebiasis.

MEDICAL ETHICS

Medical marketeering . . . If not checked, it could destroy the integrity of our profession.

—H. L. F.
in "Warning: Trained Attack Dogs on Duty"

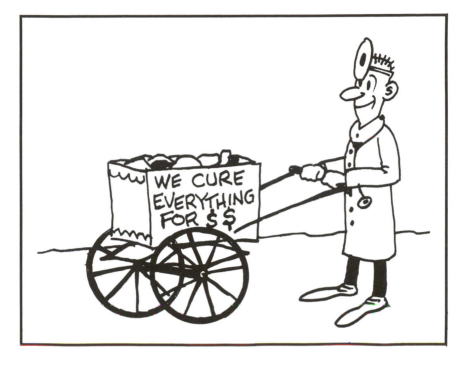

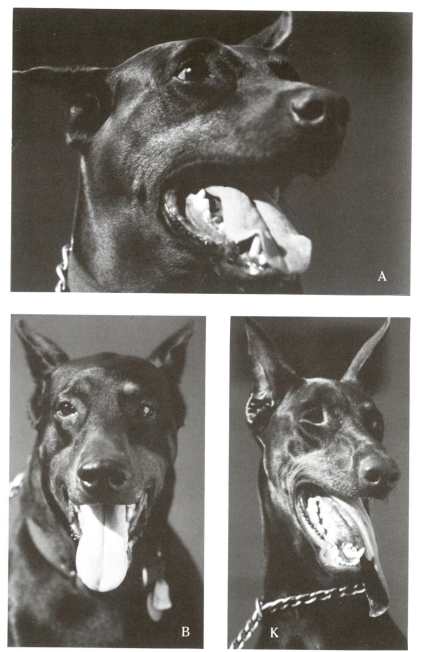

A (Autumn) + B (Baron) = K (Krysdee).
Autumn and Baron—the dogs referred to in the following article—
and their daughter, Krysdee. *(Courtesy of Dale Marks.)*

WARNING: TRAINED ATTACK DOGS ON DUTY*

Sometimes you have to hit a donkey between the eyes with a 2 x 4 just to catch his attention.

I was a donkey until the night of 3 January 1982, when two teenage boys abducted and robbed me at gunpoint. They didn't harm me physically but they really opened my eyes to the growing criminal element in our society.

Spurred by that experience, I took measures to safeguard myself and my family. One step was to buy two attack-trained Dobermans and erect yard signs advertising their presence. Since then, ours is the only house on the block that burglars haven't visited.

Today, I see another threat, one that Dobermans can't protect against. Sadly, it involves members of our own ranks in concert with other factions of the health-care industry. I call it "medical marketeering." If not checked, it could destroy the integrity of our profession.

In an eloquent discussion of this matter, Relman recently wrote: "More and more practitioners are seeking profits from business arrangements with hospitals,

---

*Reprinted by permission from the *Southern Medical Journal* 1986; 79:63-64.

equipment manufacturers, and ... companies providing ambulatory health care services."[1] He decried the commercialization of our medical-care system and called for each of us to face up to the entrepreneurialism among physicians. I share his concern and join him in the belief that we can serve our patients' interests best by divorcing ourselves from financial interest in the medical marketplace.

Like the cautionary signs in my yard, a reminder from the American Medical Association should catch our attention: "Medicine is a profession, a calling, and not a business."[2]

---

[1]Relman AS: Dealing with conflicts of interest. *N Engl J Med* 313:749-51, 1985.

[2]House of Delegates of the American Medical Association: Commercialism in the practice of medicine: Report of the Board of Trustees of the AMA, June 1983.

DISHONESTY IN MEDICINE*

When dishonesty appears to work, it is difficult to argue persuasively for honesty.

—KENNETH B. CLARK

—*New York Times,* 16 February 1975

In a recent case of fraud at Harvard Medical School, a physician-researcher brazenly fabricated data. As a postscript to the affair, another Harvard researcher said, "The man could have gently faked his way through a lifetime of research and have been greatly honored. We all know scientists like that."[1]

This event refocused international attention on deceit in science, but outright faking of research findings is only part of the problem. Less obvious kinds of dishonesty are much more common. Although we recognize that dishonesty is sometimes a matter of interpretation, we still believe it to be endemic in the medical literature, in medical school and postgraduate training, and in the way we practice medicine.

---

*Reprinted by permission from the *Southern Medical Journal* 1984; 77:1221-22.

Patricia Robie is coauthor of this article.—ED.

[1]Knox R: The Harvard fraud case: where does the problem lie? *JAMA* 249:1797-1807, 1983.

Medical Literature

Dishonesty in the medical literature, aside from the type already mentioned, can take several forms.[2] Of these, only one—clear-cut plagiarism—is uniformly condemned. The remainder are harder to detect and, even if discovered, are often condoned. For example, authors may deliberately discard undesired data or simply design their studies to yield only the desired results. They may rig references, preferentially citing their own papers while ignoring relevant reports by rivals. They may steal from themselves—autoplagiarism—and submit the same material, disguised as different articles, to a number of journals. They may not take responsibility for all elements of a paper, or they may permit their names to be listed as authors although they have made no real contribution to the work reported.

Refereeing of medical writing can generate additional abuses.[3] A referee with vested interest in a particular field of research or clinical medicine may decide for or against a manuscript depending on whether it supports or contradicts the tenets he holds. He may base his decision on who did the work and where. Worst of all, he may pilfer ideas from articles he rejects.

---

[2]Manwell C, Baker CMA: Honesty in science: a partial test of a sociobiological model of the social structure of science. *Search* 12:151-60, 1981.

Ingelfinger FJ: Peer review in biomedical publication. *Am J Med* 56:686-92, 1974.

Relman AS: Lessons from the Darsee affair (Editorial). *N Engl J Med* 308:1415-17, 1983.

[3]Manwell, Baker: Honesty in science.

Ingelfinger: Peer review in biomedical publication.

Medical School and Postgraduate Training

Dishonesty here generally hides under the guise of professional etiquette. It shows up, however, as sycophancy, silence, one-upmanship, grades, and letters of recommendation.

Sycophancy, usually called brownnosing or apple-polishing, flourishes in academia. It is particularly noticeable on teaching rounds, where the instructor and student say and do what each presumes the other wants rather than what is needed. Both can leave these sessions with ego intact—and ignorance undented.

Silence is the response of many students, house officers, and experienced physicians to a colleague whom they know or suspect to be emotionally disturbed, a substance abuser, or just plain incompetent. Their reluctance to get involved is equally deplorable when they know or suspect an associate to be cheating on an exam or lying about a case.

One-upmanship becomes dishonest when teachers and students alike intentionally spew forth untraceable information: "A group in Scandinavia first described that treatment some time ago in one of the clinical journals," or "I've seen several cases that prove my point."

Grades often reflect more a vote for the person's charisma than a rating of academic accomplishments. No one ever fails, and almost everyone is "very good" or "exceptional."[4]

Letters of recommendation rarely tell the whole truth. They typically dwell only on the positives and usually attempt to make mediocrity appear "above average."[5]

---

[4]Friedman RB: Fantasy land. *N Engl J Med* 308:651-53, 1983.

[5]Ibid.

Yager J, Strauss GD, Tardiff K: The quality of deans' letters from medical schools. *J Med Educ* 59:471-78, 1984.

Medical Practice

Dishonesty in medical practice can be difficult to spot because the manifestations characteristically conform to the "accepted standard of medical care in the community." Their common denominator is the shirking of responsibility, which compromises the perpetrator's integrity. The consequent buck-passing results in a host of ill-advised activities, including excessive consultations, inappropriate testing, undocumented diagnoses, overprescribing of medications, uncalled-for operations, needlessly prolonged hospitalizations, and unnecessary office visits. It also encourages the physician to conceal complications,[6] expurgating his medical records to prevent peer review or lawsuit.

Other acts of medical dishonesty deserve comment. Fraudulent claims relating to Medicare and Medicaid reimbursement continue to be uncovered. Hospitalizing patients solely because their insurance will not pay for a workup in the office has been common. Certain physicians, attracted by high remuneration and perhaps by the desire for public recognition, serve as expert witnesses even though they are unqualified for the role.[7]

What causes dishonesty in medicine? Two synergistic factors are paramount. One is a background of intense competition. We compete to get into medical school; we compete to stay there; we compete for the internship and residency of our choice; and thereafter we compete for patients, research grants, or whatever. The other factor is

---

[6]Goldwyn RM: Reporting or hiding a complication (Editorial). *Plast Reconstr Surg* 71:843-44, 1983.

[7]Brent RL: The irresponsible expert witness: a failure of biomedical graduate education and professional accountability. *Pediatrics* 70:754-62, 1982.

human frailty—in particular, ignorance, greed, fear of being wrong, and the need for aggrandizement. Patients frequently foster our frailties by conferring godlike qualities on us. In return, we prevaricate to protect this image for them as well as for our colleagues and ourselves.

Is there a cure? There is, but only insofar as we are willing to be role models of integrity and honesty for each other. Condoning or forgiving dishonesty of any type is itself dishonest—and, in medicine, can be tragic.

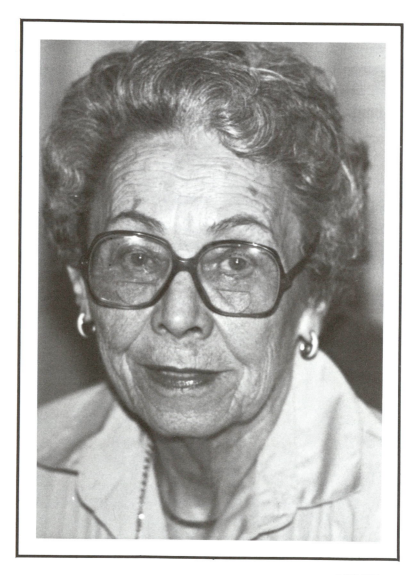

HELEN

Helen*

When the righteous die, even the Heavens cry.
—YIDDISH EXPRESSION

On the day of her funeral, it rained.

When she was a little girl, Helen recited two lines in a school play: "I have *always* been beautiful. It was *you* who could not grasp it." Throughout her life, she jokingly repeated those lines with a wry smile and turned-up nose, usually in response to statements such as, "Gee, Mother, you look beautiful today."

The fact is, Helen, my mother, really was beautiful, both physically and in the way she lived. I never saw her sulk, show prejudice, or carry a grudge. While my father was a charitable, outgoing, prominent figure in the community, Mother was his quiet, ever-supporting mate who comfortably allowed him the limelight. Her chief satisfaction came from nurturing her family. She set high standards, taught us to meet them, and let us know she loved us, even when we fell short.

After Dad died, Mother lived alone. She enjoyed maintaining her home, dining out regularly with friends,

---

*Reprinted by permission from the *Southern Medical Journal* 1986; 79:1135-36.

keeping a weekly appointment at the beauty parlor, and talking long distance with her brother and sister every Sunday morning. She liked to travel, read novels, and root for the Dallas Cowboys. Her biggest pleasure, however, was having me and my sister back home for visits.

At age eighty, Mother took part in a drama that was real. Though she had no lines, she held her audience's attention for eleven days and nights. The stage was the hospital where I am director of medical education, and the cast included me, my sister, and the others involved in Mother's care.

Three years earlier, Mother had begun having intermittent trouble speaking—as if mush were in her mouth. The episodes would disappear almost as quickly as they came on. An extensive workup identified no cause, but Mother knew that such attacks could be harbingers of a stroke, a fate she dreaded. "When my time comes, I want to go quickly. Don't let me suffer or linger," she said emphatically and often.

One day Mother phoned to say she missed me and wanted to see me. Because I had a busy schedule and could not leave town easily, Mother chose to visit me. Waiting at the airport to board the plane, she had one of her spells. But she was determined to make the trip, and she completed the flight in good spirits.

In the evening of our second day together, shortly after Mother had fixed bread pudding, my favorite dessert, it happened. Suddenly she couldn't speak; she could only make sounds. And this time the difficulty wouldn't go away. Terrified, Mother hugged me tightly and for one fleeting moment was able to say, "I love you." Within hours she lapsed into coma.

Several days later, the brutal extent of damage became evident. A massive pontine infarction (substantiated by serial CT scans) had rendered Mother irrevocably paralyzed from the eyes down. Even worse, she had regained consciousness. She was aware of her abject helplessness and could communicate with us only by blinking. She was locked in and we were locked out and there was no key.

Mother's hopeless situation raised questions that I struggled with under circumstances intensely personal and painfully sad. Which therapeutic approach is most humane for a previously independent, elderly woman who will never move or speak again but whose mind remains intact? What do you say to her when she looks at you?

I found no clear-cut answers. Indeed, the medical literature says nothing about the emotional devastation or the ethical dilemmas peculiar to the locked-in syndrome.

Initially, I told Mother that she couldn't speak because of the tube in her throat. I avoided mentioning her paralysis and anything else that might increase her fears. But as time passed, I realized that words could not fool her nor could they hide the totality of her affliction. So I limited my conversation with her to "I love you" and hoped that holding her hand, stroking her brow, and kissing her cheek would make both of us feel better.

I knew that as long as Mother remained conscious, she was experiencing severe emotional distress— distress, I think, far greater than most people ever experience. Impelled by her wish not to suffer and tormented by the sight of her suffering, I begged to have her senses dulled. Her primary physician discussed the matter with clergy, family, and colleagues and concluded, "Helen's emotional pain must be horrible, and I feel justified in relieving it."

With the medication, Mother lost the terrible awareness of her situation. I was thankful for that. But she also lost all human contact, and so I lost her.

From that point on, we made certain that Mother had good skin care, an adequate airway, and water. We expected her to die soon, but her major organs continued to function normally for five more days—while we second-guessed all our decisions. Then her temperature rose to 109 F and, mercifully, she died.

Our long ordeal had several positive features. It occurred in *my* hospital, assuring Mother the best possible attention and granting me access to her any time. It forced me and my sister to keep an agonizing vigil, one that enabled us to put aside our differences and gain new love and respect for each other. It strengthened the already close ties I had with Mother's doctors, whose competence and compassion consoled me. It moved an orderly to touch my shoulder and say, "Everything's gonna' work out, Doc." And it prompted the administrator to tell me that a host of hospital personnel had benefited from seeing another side of me: the tearful, devoted, powerless son, not the clinician in control.

But mostly, I'll remember the ordeal as Mother's final gift to me—a gift that deepened my understanding of death and dying. Death can bring happiness as well as sorrow, togetherness as well as loneliness, and tranquillity as well as turmoil. And the way we die, like the way we live, can teach much and inspire many.

As we lowered Mother to rest beside Dad, the clouds broke, and I could see the sun.

A Comment on "Helen"*

Dr. Fred's poignant account in this issue tells us that at age eighty "Helen" suffered a massive pontine infarction leaving her paralyzed from the eyes down but with her mind nevertheless "intact." Her physician-son concluded rightly that she was "locked-in" but wrongly that "we were locked out." That he was not locked out, strictly speaking, is evident from his words of comfort to her, his initial reassurance that her difficulty in speaking was caused by the tube in her throat, and his decision not to mention her paralysis or "anything else that might increase her fears." He and others were "locked out" only after his decision to implement an intrusive procedure, namely, "dulling her senses," which caused her to "lose all human contact, and so I lost her." She was expected to die soon, "but her major organs continued to function normally."

Her survival with major organs functioning normally was somewhat a surprise and as a result "we second-guessed all our decisions." The two major decisions were, first, to dull Helen's senses, and second, to refrain

---

*Reprinted by permission from the *Southern Medical Journal* 1986; 79:1057-58.

from any positive therapy, although she did receive "good skin care, an adequate airway, and water." Five days later, her unexplained elevated temperature of 109 F brought an end to her life.

All this left the physician-son with "ethical dilemmas." What is the ethical problem here? There can be no question that Helen was aware of her condition, she was full of years, her eyes communicated "severe emotional distress," her condition was irreversible, as well as terminal. Moreover, she had earlier expressed a desire to go quickly "when my time comes. Don't let me suffer or linger."

What complicates the ethical issue in Helen's case is that during her massive paralysis, her mind was intact. Theoretically at least, she could listen to music, hear books read, and hear the latest exploits of her favorite Dallas Cowboys. All this was deliberately closed out to her on the plausible grounds that she was suffering a special form of pain, emotional not physical, but pain nevertheless and with no hope of improvement. In the past, serious ethical questions were raised about the justification of terminating the "life" of a brain-dead or neocortical-dead patient. Here, by contrast, the ethical question focuses upon the act of rendering an intact mind, even though "locked in," dysfunctional. To solve whose problem?

In a current similar case, another physician-son resents the active measures of the medical team on behalf of his ninety-six-year-old mother, saying that "since the preservation of her life helps no one, and is desired neither by her nor those who love her most dearly, why could her doctors not be content to let her die in peace and serenity? Why did they pursue a vigorous therapy that could benefit no one except their own satisfaction in thwarting death, regardless of the consequences?" She continues to live even though "she has lost her functional and mental independence," leading her physician-son to say, "I weep for my mother and for what has happened to my profession."[1]

What has happened to "my profession" is that physicians are reluctant to terminate either actively or passively a person's life deliberately and as a matter of public policy. So strong is the ethical requirement to preserve life that even in this extremity the decision to cease all therapy does not come easily. In Helen's case, the reluctance to await a more natural end raises an even more acute ethical problem inasmuch as an intact mind is turned off the way a candle is blown out. Neither the earlier request not to linger nor the obvious decline in the quality of life is sufficient to overcome the fundamental claim to life of an intact mind. For this reason, even terminal cancer patients are frequently given only enough medication to reduce or eliminate their physical pain but not so much as to obliterate their consciousness. Here the circumstance is not only that the mind is locked in but that it was intact.

A celebrated case involved a noted physician in his late forties who endured the gradual ravages of amyotrophic lateral sclerosis, an affliction distinguished in several ways from Helen's but whose end stage involves the locked-in syndrome.[2] Ironically, this physician-patient's earlier specialty was neurology, which of course meant that he was completely aware of the unfolding of his textbooklike case of ALS. Despite his quadriplegia and bulbar symptoms followed by wasting

---

[1]Feinstein AR: The state of the art. *JAMA* 255:1488, 1986.

[2]Rabin PL, Rabin D: *To Provide Safe Passage: The Humanistic Aspects of Medicine.* New York, Philosophical Library, 1985.

of the tongue, dysarthria, dysphonia, and dysphagia, his mind was intact. He derived special joy from listening to music even while he and his physician-wife grieved over the multiple and continuing losses of various functions. For him, and them, the presence of consciousness was of the essence—that is what made him a person and that is what neither he nor his family wished to interrupt intrusively. Although they did not use moral language to describe their determination to sustain his life, they instinctively arrived at the ethical principle that human life is to be preserved as long as there is consciousness and cognitive function in contrast to a vegetative state or a condition of neocortical death.[3]

—Samuel E. Stumpf, Ph.D.
Research Professor of Medical Philosophy
Department of Medicine
Vanderbilt University School of Law

---

[3]Ibid.

"HELEN" REVISITED*

Rhadames, lately the much lauded conquering hero and once commander of the pharaoh's armies, is convicted of high treason and condemned to die by being entombed alive in the crypt beneath the Temple of Ptah. In one of the most moving scenes in all opera, amidst the chanting of the priests and the wails of the pharaoh's daughter Amneris, Aïda, the Ethiopian princess, quietly joins her lover in his entombment; presumably, somewhere down the line, they die ecstatically in each other's arms. It is all very romantic—but do they? It obviously is well that the opera leave them there. Real life does not make things so convenient.

There are all sorts of horror tales of people being buried alive, both accidentally and deliberately. In our modern-day attention to the ritual of burial, embalming obviates the former possibility, but it has not always been so and with increasing costs may not always be either. Too, people are buried as buildings collapse or as mines cave in. If they survive, they are doubtlessly plagued by nightmares forever after. Most people have

*Reprinted by permission from the *Southern Medical Journal* 1986; 79:1055-56.

likely considered, at one time or another, the possibility that something like that might happen to them. Most shrug—or perhaps better, shudder—the notion off; a few become obsessed with it. Either way, it is not pleasant to contemplate.

With modern technology having made it possible increasingly to delay the day of reckoning as our mortal bodies refuse to support life any longer, the reams that have been written about the right to die are as the stars of the sky or the sands of the seashore. Equally as much has been written about its antithesis, the right to life (which might more properly be called the right *of* life). Armies of philosophers have waxed eloquent on both sides of the question. The courts have decided, perhaps as a temporizing measure, that "brain death"—where the electroencephalogram shows no evidence of brain activity despite a physiologically functional body—is grounds for discontinuing life-support systems. The rationale for this decision is that the person has fled his earthly shell for wherever it is that persons ultimately go, and that there is no point in using up precious resources, which include the stamina of loved ones, simply to keep a useless carcass functioning. This support can be offered indefinitely, and has been. We no longer must.

What does one do, though, when that carcass, though physiologically functional, refuses any longer to obey its owner, entrapping the person therein? It is as if one were forever locked inside a parked automobile, with no possibility of moving the car or getting out of it—in short, being entombed alive. Not much has been said about that. Of the two, it seems much the worse, does it not? In the first case, the person is gone; we have no control over his destination. We can move the car and be done with it. In the second, however, we are stuck with an occupied automobile, which we can either leave where it is or destroy it, but we cannot free its occupant. Do we then leave it and block off that parking place as no longer available to any others, or do we free it up by towing the car away and pushing it, with its occupant, into a hole?

We find ourselves in the situation of the man who, when asked in exasperation by his nagging wife whether he was a man or a mouse, desperately asked if there wasn't something in between. Some years ago, in a movie entitled *Soylent Green,* aged individuals tired of living were helped out of this world painlessly in pleasant surroundings amidst soft music of their own choosing and pastoral scenes projected on the walls; in short, euthanasia at its best. The trouble with that solution is that it is acceptable as neither a legal, a moral, nor an ethical choice for either the patient or his doctors.

A touching piece entitled simply "Helen," published on page 1135 of this issue, suggests a possible middle position. Helen, buried alive in her useless, unresponsive body, was through drugs assisted halfway out of it into a dream world until natural forces completed the process. She was freed without being killed—a pseudo brain death, so to speak. A commentary on the piece (page 1057) points out problems arising from such a course and suggests that though the solution seems satisfactory enough, that still is no simple solution.

The pointed question asked in the commentary, "To solve whose problem?" is one with which Helen's physician-son had struggled desperately. Though there are similarities, there is also a difference between Helen's situation and that of the Drs. Rabin, referred to by Dr. Stumpf, that we must recognize. As David Rabin's faculties progressively failed, he and his wife—having full knowledge of the course his disease would take—made the choice to stay together to the end, devising intricate means for him to communicate with her and even to author papers when he could move no more than an eyelash. It was a gradually progressive thing, and for them infinitely better than brain death. Helen, though, had this cataclysm thrust upon her suddenly. Terror would be the only natural reaction. Once that terror subsided, however, how might that acute mind have grappled with it? The mind has the power to turn itself off in situations it cannot handle. It also has incredible power to adapt.

I had an aunt who until she died just short of her hundredth birthday had a complete, active set of mental faculties and until the last couple of years was also a spry elder citizen who lived alone, under the watchful eye of a daughter, in the home where she had reared her five children. For those last years she was confined to her room, able only to sit up in a chair by the window. Not long before she died she told me that she didn't know why the Lord had kept her around for so long—"To pray for the rest of you, I guess," she said.

It is easy to consider all these things in retrospect, particularly when one is not intimately involved. We owe Dr. Fred a debt of gratitude for having the courage to bare his soul for our benefit. It is the only way we can learn to cope with the dilemmas thrust upon us by modern technology. Outside the parked, locked car the world goes by. Its windows are clean, and the radio works. We are locked in, but even though we are locked in and cannot be participants in it, the world is not locked out. Is that enough?

If drugs are used simply to close out the world and not end life, as in Helen's case, the situation can, if contemplation demands, be easily reversed. For her, death made the decision with hyperthermia, apparently of central origin. Some might say she was called home to spare her and her loved ones further anguish.

When we gained the power to wrest concessions from death as an enemy, we lost the right to invite him in as a friend. In trying to have it both ways, to usurp power that is not ours, we have become entrapped in a moral morass. Once again, man's reach has exceeded his grasp. No matter how much we might wish it otherwise, we are not allowed life on our own terms.

—John B. Thomison, MD
Editor

—AND MORE

*Stupidity is essentially God-given; ignorance is clearly
man-made. We are only as ignorant as we choose to be.*

—H. L. F.
— in "Stupid, or Ignorant?"

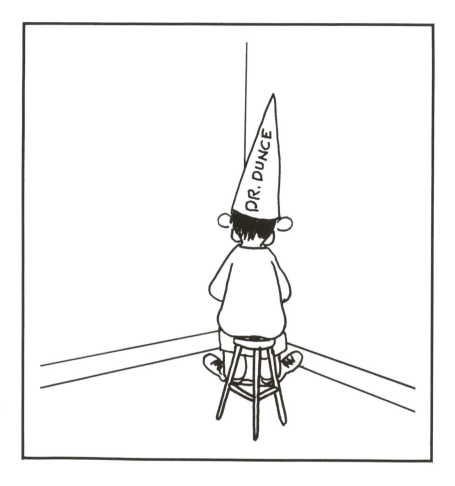

STUPID, OR IGNORANT?*

Everyone is ignorant, only on different subjects.
—WILL ROGERS

Stupid and *ignorant* are words we use almost daily. Though we often use them interchangeably, we shouldn't.

Stupid refers to slow-wittedness. Stupidity can be either inherited or the result of a diseased brain, a blow to the head, the effects of drugs, or the like. Thus, most stupid people are stupid through no fault of their own. And, unfortunately, they can do little to prevent their affliction or improve their lot.

Ignorant denotes a lack of knowledge. Fortunately, the depth and duration of ignorance are inversely proportional to the effort one makes to become knowledgeable. Yet the most learned person remains profoundly ignorant of many things.

The point is this: no specific remedy exists for stupidity, but education uniformly cures ignorance. Viewed another way—stupidity is essentially God-given; ignorance is clearly man-made. We are only as ignorant as we choose to be.

---

*Reprinted by permission from *Houston Medical Journal* 1985; 1:51.

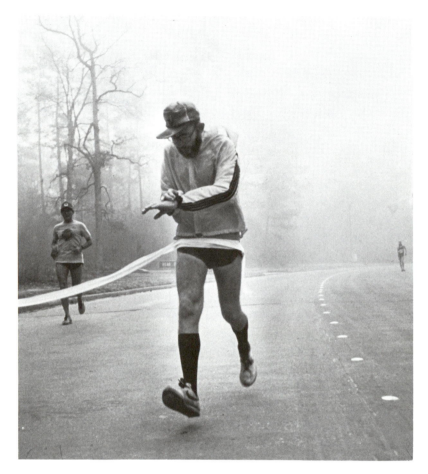

The author goes airborne at dawn to set a national age-group record (50-54 years) for the 100-Mile Run. The Athletics Congress Gulf Association Ultramarathons, Houston, Texas, 20-21 February 1982. *(Courtesy of Michael Fred.)*

I May Be a Fanatic, But I'm a Healthy One*

I am a fifty-five-year-old physician, a specialist in internal medicine, and a running fanatic.

In 1966, I was a sedentary, overweight smoker. My only exercise was jumping to conclusions.

Dissatisfied with that existence, I decided to restructure my life-style and realign my priorities. I gave up my cigarettes, paid attention to my diet, and began to run. Since then, I've run more than 100,000 miles—20 miles a day, rain or shine, hot or cold.

Even though the health benefits of a regular exercise program are medically incontrovertible, no one needs to run twenty miles a day to be healthy. But almost anyone *could* work up to it.

In fact, I don't run high mileage just for my health. I also do it because it makes me feel better, it keeps me trim, it makes me more productive in my profession, and because I *like* to run.

---

*Copyright 1984, *USA Today,* 7 August. Reprinted with permission. Mark Scheid assisted in writing this column.

Many people seem determined to condemn strenuous exercise. Yet that attitude reveals a curious double standard.

In our society, if you toil eight hours a day at a job you don't like, it's a virtue; you're "hard working." Olympic athletes often train more than fifty hours a week to perfect their skills, and they are held up as examples of dedication and patriotism.

But when people like me spend three or four hours a day doing something that we enjoy—which helps us and hurts no one— newspapers carry editorials decrying "exercise fanatics."

Why? I think I know. My type of exercise— running— is a rather public sport, often done in parks and along roads. It is easily seen by nonexercisers.

That wouldn't matter except that most nonexercisers, I suspect, believe that they *ought* to be exercising, and at the sight of a jogger, they indict themselves for sloth.

The largest group of fanatics in this country—the fanatical nonexercisers—will use the recent death of Jim Fixx as evidence that "all that exercise doesn't really help anyway, and it's dangerous."

The medical facts belie such logic. The best way to avoid illness and protect against premature coronary artery disease is to bypass smoking, overeating, and inactivity—the kind of triple bypass therapy all of us can afford.

Being Careful Wasn't Enough*

I never thought it would happen to me. But it did. It could happen to you, too.

I'm a street-runner—always have been and, until recently, thought I always would be. I'm also a cautious street-runner. I run *against* traffic whenever possible, always obey traffic signals, assiduously avoid running at night, and never challenge a car. I run the same route virtually every day and know every detail of the traffic patterns and signal lights along the way. Yet, despite twenty-two years of running on Houston streets and covering 130,000 miles in the process, my carefulness didn't protect me from someone else's carelessness.

Being careful wasn't enough.

It happened during the afternoon rush hour on 4 June 1987 as I was crossing a busy downtown intersection about to finish my daily training run. I had crossed that intersection countless times; my office is on that corner and I run to and from that point every day.

The green light was in my favor and the "Walk" sign was on. But as I jogged toward the middle of the intersection, a young motorist coming from my left ran a

_____

*Published by permission of *Ultrarunning* 1987; 7:34-35.

red light and hit me. The next thing I knew, I was lying on the street looking skyward, noting the clouds rolling around and around at a rapid pace.

Being careful wasn't enough.

Witnesses say that the collision bent the car's front bumper and right front fender and that my head shattered the car's windshield. I clearly recall the moment of impact; it was painless. Seconds later, however, my head, neck, left shoulder, right side, and left foot began to hurt.

As I lay on the pavement, I felt irritated—because the accident would interrupt my tight schedule for a few hours and leave me with a sore body for a few days. So, to save time and trouble, I asked the ambulance attendants to take me to my office rather than to the hospital. They didn't.

Extensive x-ray exams showed no apparent broken bones and a CAT scan of my head was normal. "You've just got a concussion and a lot of bumps, bruises, and abrasions. You'll be back running in a couple of weeks," the doctors said. But as each day in the hospital passed, the pain in my head, shoulder, and right side got worse, and my left foot became more swollen and discolored. My initial feelings of irritation were giving way to fear—fear that my injuries were more serious than anyone had thought. In fact, I feared I might die.

The true extent of my injuries became evident at the end of the first week. Magnetic Resonance Imaging (MRI) detected one definite and one probable skull fracture, a blood clot on my brain, and multiple hemorrhages into both front halves of my brain. Follow-up x-rays also identified subtle fractures of my left scapula, right rib cage, and left foot, along with partial dislocation of my cervical spine. Because of the brain damage, I had lost my sense of taste and smell. Because of the spinal damage, I had to wear a neck brace night and day. After eleven days in the hospital, I went home.

Being careful wasn't enough.

Now, two months after the accident, my wife drives me to my office and back every day. I won't be permitted to drive until MRI shows resolution of the blood clot and hemorrhages affecting my brain. I still wear the neck brace; whether I'll need an operation on my neck is unsettled. My sense of taste has returned, but my sense of smell remains decreased. Otherwise, I have no neurological and no visual impairment. I try to maintain some degree of conditioning by riding a stationary bike daily.

As I ponder my future several questions keep recurring. When I recover sufficiently, should my chief form of exercise be running, or should it be walking, cycling, or swimming? If I choose to run only (and I probably will), should I try to regain my previous ultramarathon fitness, or should I set less strenuous goals? Should I compete or just run for fun? Should I run on the streets again, or would I be wiser to run on a track or bike path?

Regardless of what happens, I don't feel angry or sorry for myself. I feel very fortunate to be alive and apparently free of any long-term disability.

Being careful wasn't enough—I had to be lucky, too.

To Be "B" or Not to Be "B"?*

Are you intensely ambitious? Do you have a strong competitive drive? Are you constantly preoccupied with deadlines? If so, your personality is Type A. If you lack these traits, your personality is Type B. The difference may be important—or it may not.

In 1959 Friedman and Rosenman reported that people with Type A personality had a sevenfold greater prevalence of clinical coronary artery disease than did those with Type B personality.[1] Since then, many conflicting reports have appeared concerning the relationship between Type A personality and the development and progression of coronary artery disease.[2]

Four years ago, the National Institutes of Health sponsored a panel to review the available data on this

---

*Reprinted by permission from *Houston Medical Journal* 1985; 1:135-36.

[1]Friedman M, Rosenman RH: Association of specific overt behavior pattern with blood and cardiovascular findings. Blood cholesterol level, blood clotting time, incidence of arcus senilis, and clinical coronary artery disease. *JAMA* 169:1286-96, 1959.

[2]Case RB, Heller SS, Case NB, et al.: Type A behavior and survival after acute myocardial infarction. *N Engl J Med* 312:737-41, 1985.

matter.[3] The panel concluded that Type A behavior constituted an independent risk factor for coronary artery disease. The risk was similar in magnitude to that created by smoking, hypercholesterolemia, or elevated systolic blood pressure. More recently, Case et al. (who are members of the Multicenter Post-Infarction Research Group) argued that "there is no uniform evidence to substantiate either a close relation between the characteristic behavior of the Type A personality and coronary artery disease or the protective effects of the Type B personality."[4]

The controversy is continuing. Friedman and his group are now altering Type A behavior in patients who have had a heart attack.[5] They say that such alteration is associated with a significant reduction of subsequent nonfatal myocardial infarctions.

But is it necessarily good to change Type A behavior? The change could mean "demotion in job status, in job function, in the regard of colleagues and possibly in personal income."[6] Therefore, if we feel the need to alter

---

[3]The Review Panel on Coronary-Prone Behavior and Coronary Heart Disease: Coronary-prone behavior and coronary heart disease. A critical review. *Circulation* 63:1199-1215, 1981.

[4]Case, Heller, Case: Type A behavior.

[5]Friedman M, Thoresen CE, Gill JJ, et al.: Feasibility of altering type A behavior pattern after myocardial infarction. Recurrent coronary prevention project study: Methods, baseline results and preliminary findings. *Circulation* 66:83-92, 1982.

Friedman M, Thoresen CE, Gill JJ, et al.: Alteration of type A behavior and reduction in cardiac recurrences in postmyocardial infarction patients. *Am Heart J* 108:237-48, 1984.

[6]Editorial: Are we killing ourselves or not? *Lancet* 2:669-70, 1981.

someone's behavior, why don't we convert a few of the B's into A's? All things considered, the world just might be better off.

FEELING SORRY FOR OURSELVES*

From time to time we all feel sorry for ourselves. To illustrate, I offer the following story:

In May 1978 I went to Honolulu to compete in a 100-kilometer (62.1-mile) run. The race began just after dark under junglelike conditions—hot, humid, and still. The starters soon became widely separated on the dimly lit, four-mile loop. In the middle of the night, when I was tired, wanted to quit, and ached all over, especially in my legs, I came up on a particularly slow runner. I decided to stay by his side for a while because the slower pace was a welcome relief. I complained bitterly to him about how miserable I felt and how much my legs hurt. He, in turn, listened attentively and offered words of encouragement, but said nothing of feeling bad himself. After a bit, I picked up the pace and left him behind.

I came up on him again at sunrise. In the light of day, I had my first opportunity to get a good look at him. To my astonishment and dismay, he had an artificial leg.

One year later I returned to Honolulu for a 100-mile race, bringing along five people to help me during the projected 20-hour ordeal. We were setting up my special

---

*Reprinted by permission from *Houston Medical Journal* 1985; 1:87.

food and other supplies near the starting line when I saw my friend making similar preparations. He had no support crew, but he did have some very special equipment: three spare legs.

If anyone had a right to feel sorry for himself, this man did. But whatever he felt, he didn't give in or give up. He did the best he could with what he had. Do we?

SOMEBODY DID MY JOB*

My goal in this column is always to offer something easy to read, easy to digest, enjoyable, and yet informative. That's difficult, as everybody knows. Though almost anybody could assume this task from time to time, nobody else really should. This time, however, somebody else did.

A Little Story

This is a little story about four people named Everybody, Somebody, Anybody, and Nobody. An important job had to be done, and Everybody was sure that Somebody would do it. Anybody could have done it, but Nobody did it. Somebody got angry about that, because it was Everybody's job. Everybody thought Anybody could do it, but Nobody realized that Everybody wouldn't do it. It ended up that Everybody blamed Somebody when Nobody did what Anybody could have done!

— ANONYMOUS

Thank you, Somebody, for doing my job.

---

*Reprinted by permission from *Houston Medical Journal* 1988; 4:3.

NO ONE IS PERFECT*

Andy Rooney makes a fortune complaining about life's ups and downs. He usually paints his problems with a brush of humor, but at the moment they occur, he probably isn't amused.

Well, I'm no Andy Rooney, and I don't get paid for complaining. Furthermore, when things upset me, my response is not ordinarily funny. But I'm going to complain anyway about a "funny" disparity—the way society views malpractice.

When I hire an individual or company to do a job—repair my fence, install my refrigerator, move my household furnishings, service my car—inferior work and recurrent delays are common, *if* the "care provider" shows up at all. The persons responsible for these fiascoes offer the usual excuses but rarely give satisfactory explanations. They also seem oblivious to the inconvenience and distress their incompetence generates. To make matters worse, they fully expect me to forgive, even condone, their mistakes. "After all," they say, "no one is perfect."

*Reprinted by permission from the *Southern Medical Journal* 1989; 82:1.

Yet when these same individuals seek medical help, they expect perfection. They expect a specific diagnosis. They expect a cure. With anything less, they are more inclined to sue than forgive. Why this disparity, this inequity, this injustice?

"Because doctors deal with our lives," they say, "and that's much more important than losing office files or failing to fix a leaky radiator."

Yes, the practice of medicine *is* important, and our responsibility is awesome. But I believe doctors try hard to meet that responsibility. I believe, too, that the public generally views physician error as malpractice while viewing its own malpractices as mere human frailties. Of course, you may not agree with me or I may not have made myself clear.

But then, no one is perfect.

THE JOURNEY TO THE GRAVE*

We eat too much,
drink too much, smoke
too much, drive too fast,
and walk too little.[1]

—MARGARET C. HEAGARTY, M.D.
National Academy of Sciences

From the moment we are born, each of us literally begins a journey to the grave. Although the trek inevitably ends, many factors may influence its quality and duration. One such factor is exercise.

Certain beneficial effects of exercise are well established. These include improved cardiac function, lowered blood pressure, reduced fasting and postprandial hyperlipidemia, decreased blood glucose levels, increased plasma fibrinolytic activity, slowed platelet aggregation, and loss of weight if caloric intake stays constant.

Whether exercise delays or prevents the onset of coronary artery disease remains arguable. In fact, this

---

*Reprinted by permission from the *Medical Journal of St. Joseph Hospital* 1980; 15:91-94.

[1]Heagarty MC: Life-style change—A difficult challenge. *Pediatrics* 58:314, 1976.

question may never be answered because the problem is so complex. Nevertheless, two scientific studies in particular have provided evidence that a physically active life-style diminishes the risk of myocardial infarction.

First, Paffenbarger and his colleagues investigated 3,263 longshoremen over a sixteen-year period, giving special emphasis to deaths from coronary artery disease and stroke.[2] They correlated such deaths with the degree of physical activity, amount of cigarette smoking, level of blood pressure, and weight-for-height pattern. They found that cargo-handlers, who daily expend nearly 1,000 more calories than other longshoremen, had a coronary death rate 25% lower than that of their more sedentary work companions (i.e., fifty-nine versus eighty per 10,000 man-years of experience). The coronary death rate remained lower for the cargo-handlers even when their smoking habits, blood pressure, and weight varied. By contrast, the death rates from stroke were similar among cargo-handlers and less active longshoremen (i.e., fourteen and sixteen per 10,000 man-years of experience respectively). These findings suggest that physical activity has a more striking influence on myocardial infarction than on atherosclerosis per se.

The second investigation, by Mann et al., involved the Masai tribe of East Africa.[3] The Masai live almost exclusively on meat and fermented milk. Their young men consume about 300 gm of fat and 500 mg of cholesterol daily, an intake of animal fat exceeding that

----

[2]Paffenbarger RS Jr, Laughlin ME, Gima AS, Black RA: Work activity of longshoremen as related to death from coronary heart disease and stroke. *N Engl J Med* 282:1109, 1970.

[3]Mann GV, Spoerry A, Gray M, Jarashow D: Atherosclerosis in the Masai. *Am J Epidemiol* 95:26, 1972.

of American men. The Masai, however, are exceptionally active and physically fit. Of 600 Masai examined, including 350 men older than forty years of age, only one man had unequivocal electrocardiographic evidence of myocardial infarction. High blood pressure was unusual and serum cholesterol levels were low, rarely exceeding 150 mg per 100 ml; neither rose with age.

Mann and his associates also collected at autopsy the hearts and aortas of fifty Masai men. All of the men had died suddenly, the majority from trauma or infection. None had died of heart disease. Half were forty years of age or older. The aortas showed extensive lipid infiltration and fibrous changes; only a few had obstructing lesions. Although the coronary arteries displayed intimal thickening equal to that of elderly men in America, the vessels had enlarged with age to more than compensate for the associated atherosclerosis. The authors speculated that the Masai's physical fitness caused their coronary arteries to become more capacious, thereby protecting them from the consequences of atherosclerosis. Put another way, this study suggests that exercise can override the deleterious vascular effects of a fatty diet.

Once someone decides to begin exercising, which sport or activity should he choose? The choice depends in part on what the person enjoys doing and what his goals are. In this regard, the accompanying tables should be helpful.

One final inarguable point—regular exercise, regardless of its type, induces a sense of well-being that only those "who have been there" can truly appreciate. Admittedly, millions of people feel fine without any sort of planned physical activity. They would feel better, however, if they adopted an exercise program. Indeed, "for both the ill and the healthy, a vigorous physical activity pattern seems to confer manifold advantages for the mind, body, and possibly most importantly, the spirit."[4]

Epilogue

In 1966 I weighed 200 lbs., ate three large meals a day, smoked cigarettes and cigars, and drank a few cocktails before dinner. My only exercise was jumping to conclusions. Dissatisfied with that existence, I decided to restructure my life-style and realign my priorities.

Now, I run 120 miles or more a week, eat only one meal a day, do not smoke or drink, and weigh 150 lbs. Although I felt good before the change, I feel much better today. I am happier, remain alert longer, and rarely get tired.

Thus, fourteen years ago I made a decision. That decision may not have added years to my life, but it *has* added life to my years. And it has made *my* journey more fulfilling.

----

[4]Bortz WM II: Effect of exercise on aging—Effect of aging on exercise. *J Am Geriatrics Soc* 28:49, 1980.

WHAT KINDS OF EXERCISE BEST PROMOTE PHYSICAL FITNESS?

	Jogging	Bicycling	Swimming	Skating (ice or roller)	Handball/Squash	Skiing (Nordic)	Skiing (Alpine)	Basketball	Tennis	Calisthenics	Walking	Golf*	Softball	Bowling
Physical Fitness														
Cardiorespiratory endurance (stamina)	21	19	21	18	19	19	16	19	16	10	13	8	6	5
Muscular endurance	20	18	20	17	18	19	18	17	16	13	14	8	8	5
Muscular strength	17	16	14	15	15	15	15	15	14	16	11	9	7	5
Flexibility	9	9	15	13	16	14	14	13	14	19	7	8	9	7
Balance	17	18	12	20	17	16	21	16	16	15	8	8	7	6
General Well-Being														
Weight control	21	20	15	17	19	17	15	19	16	12	13	6	7	5
Muscle definition	14	15	14	14	11	12	14	13	13	18	11	6	5	5
Digestion	13	12	13	11	13	12	9	10	12	11	11	7	8	7
Sleep	16	15	16	15	12	15	12	12	11	12	14	6	7	6
Totals	148	142	140	140	140	139	134	134	128	126	102	66*	64	51

*Ratings for golf are based on the fact that many Americans use a golf cart or caddy. If the golfer walks the links, the physical fitness value moves up appreciably.

In a study by the President's Council on Physical Fitness, seven medical experts rated fourteen popular forms of exercise in relation to physical fitness. Ratings were on a scale of 0 to 3; a cumulative rating of 21 indicated maximum benefit. Ratings were based on regular participation (at least four times a week) and vigorous activity (at least a half hour each time). The intensity of the exercise was crucial to the ratings, and the panelists assumed that the individual would exert maximum effort. (Data reprinted from "How Different Sports Rate in Promoting Physical Fitness," in *Resident and Staff Physician*, August 1976, pages 43-50, with permission of the publisher.)

• RELATIONSHIP OF CALORIES TO VARIOUS ACTIVITIES •

PORTION OF FOOD	APPROX* CALORIES	APPROXIMATE NUMBER OF CALORIES EXPENDED IN TIME SHOWN FOR EACH ACTIVITY† [0:00.00 = hours:minutes.fractions]				
		Reclining 80 cal/hr	Walking 310 cal/hr	Bicycling 490 cal/hr	Swimming 670 cal/hr	Running 1165 cal/hr
1 tsp granulated sugar	15	0:12	0:03	0:02	0:01.5	0:00.75
1 pat marg/butter	50	0:38	0:10	0:06	0:04.5	0:02.5
½ medium grapefruit	55	0:42	0:11	0:07	0:05	0:03
½ cup orange juice	55	0:42	0:11	0:07	0:05	0:03
1 slice white bread	60	0:46	0:12	0:07	0:05	0:03
1 medium apple	70	0:54	0:13	0:08	0:06	0:04
1 large egg	80	1:01	0:15	0:10	0:07	0:04
1 cup skim milk	90	1:10	0:17	0:11	0:08	0:05
1 tbsp peanut butter	95	1:15	0:18	0:12	0:08.5	0:05
8 oz cola beverage	95	1:15	0:18	0:12	0:08.5	0:05
2 slices crisp bacon	100	1:17	0:19	0:12	0:09	0:05
1 ounce process cheddar cheese	105	1:21	0:20	0:13	0:09	0:05
1 doughnut	125	1:35	0:24	0:15	0:11	0:06
12 ounces beer	150	1:55	0:29	0:18	0:13	0:08
1 frankfurter	155	1:59	0:30	0:19	0:14	0:08
1 cup whole milk	160	2:05	0:31	0:20	0:14	0:08
3 ounces broiled hamburger, lean	185	2:25	0:36	0:23	0:17	0:10
3 ounces broiled hamburger, reg	245	3:10	0:47	0:30	0:22	0:13

*Source: "Nutritive Value of Foods," Home and Garden Bulletin no. 72, United States Department of Agriculture, rev. 1964.

†Calorie expenditure rates are those used by Frank Konishi, Ph.D., in "Food Energy Equivalents of Various Activities" (*Journal of the American Dietetic Association,* 46:186-88, March 1965) and pertain to an "average" 70 kg (154 lb) male. Heavier individuals will use calories at a higher rate, lighter individuals at a lower rate.

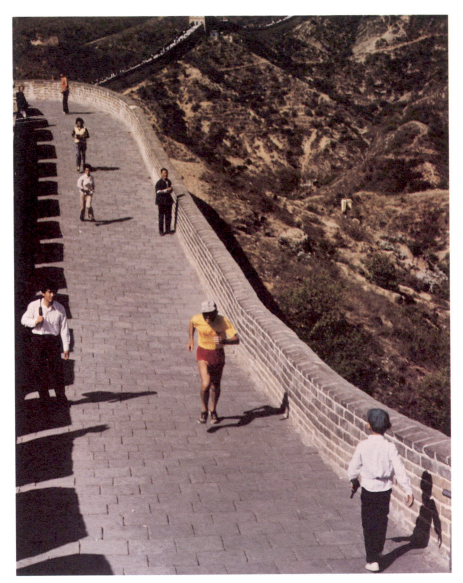

The author running on the Great Wall of China, 13 May 1984.

RUNNING THROUGH CHINA*
A HOUSTON DOCTOR EXPLORES
THE PEOPLE'S REPUBLIC ON FOOT

Editor's note: Dr. Herbert L. Fred, director of medical education at St. Joseph Hospital, toured China for two weeks last May with a group composed primarily of physicians. They visited medical facilities in several major cities, exchanged lectures and information with Chinese colleagues, and went sightseeing. A seasoned runner, Dr. Fred, fifty-five, took to the streets in his free time.

The sidewalks look like the start of the Boston and New York Marathons, each block teeming with people, shoulder to shoulder, some just standing around, others walking aimlessly about. Unlike people in marathons, however, everybody here appears the same size and shape, has the same color of hair and skin, and wears the same getup— blue pants, blue jacket, blue cap. Now pack the streets with millions of bicycles, and you have the scene that greets our tour group in every Chinese city we visit.

During a two-week trip last May, sightseeing activities for the group taught me a lot about China. But by squeezing in some early-morning runs and going where tour buses never go, I learned a great deal more.

---

*Reprinted by permission from *Houston Post Magazine,* 28 October 1984, pp. 13, 14, 22.

Our first stop was Shanghai, but I didn't run there; the day before leaving the States, I had injured my knee in a twenty-four-hour race. If I had to forgo running anywhere in China, however, Shanghai was the place to do so; it took the prize for congestion. And from dawn to dusk, bus horns blared incessantly at the intrepid cyclists.

Leaving Shanghai, my group took the train to Wuxi, a major manufacturing center for clay figurines and silk. Splitting the city is The Grand Canal, a 1200-mile-long, 1400-year-old, busy, man-made waterway. Our hotel was located on the outskirts of the town near a large lake and rolling hills where traffic flowed freely. The setting was too inviting to resist. With my knee almost well, I ran for the first time in China along that lake. An American engineer and his wife accompanied me, and we were the only runners in sight.

I arose early the next day, eager to get in another run. At 4:40 A.M., however, I found the hotel lobby empty and dark, its front doors locked. So I ran up and down a dimly lit, adjacent corridor until an employee showed up at 5:00 A.M. and opened the doors. Once outside, I discovered that the hotel gates were also locked, but I was able to persuade the sleepy guard to let me through. Subsequently, I learned that our hotel in Shanghai had been locked from 11:00 P.M. to 5:00 A.M. daily, a procedure to be repeated in Xi'an as well. In response to my inquiry, the Chinese guide said that locking our hotels kept undesirables out, but I viewed it as keeping the occupants in.

The following day I begged off from my group and devoted the morning to a long, leisurely run on a narrow asphalt road that soon became gravel, then dirt. Sharing the road with me were occasional cyclists, dilapidated buses, and antiquated tractors, but no cars or runners. Moving through lush farmland and several small communities, I passed a slew of villagers, most of whom stopped their chores to stare at me as I jogged by. Many smiled, some waved, and several youngsters said "Hallow." Surprisingly, I saw only a few dogs, cats, chickens, ducks, and goats, and no horses, cattle, or pigs. I had expected to see many dogs and cats in the country because the government outlaws them in the cities, reputedly to reduce filth and disease.

After running about eight miles into the hills, I came across a military compound surrounded by high stone walls with huge iron gates. Soldiers were everywhere— one-third of them women—all dressed in olive-green uniforms with red stars in the center of their olive-green Mao caps. Interestingly, their shoes varied considerably—from oxfords and loafers to beat-up sneakers. The soldiers were all on foot and none carried guns. Deciding not to push my luck, I turned back quickly, waving nonchalantly and saying "Ni hao" (how do you do) to the soldiers. Down the road I met a convoy of army trucks and motorcycles. Two policemen with the convoy motioned me to stop, and I did. As they walked toward me, thoughts of prolonged interrogation and possible imprisonment flashed through my mind. Oddly, however, I felt intrigued, not scared. I welcomed the adventure that was unfolding.

They talked to me in Chinese, but all I could do was point to a badge that contained my name and that of the tour agency. As the policemen recorded the information in a little red book, they called out each letter of my name in English, suggesting that they could have spoken to me in English. Then, after about five minutes of discussion between themselves, they let me go. They followed me on bicycles, however, for the next five miles. When I had clearly exited their territory, they turned away. The next day I ran a different course.

From Wuxi we traveled by train to Nanjing (Nanking), where life moves at a slower pace. Towering trees arching over the streets and lovely parks made this the prettiest city on our tour. Running in Nanjing opened new vistas of China for me. I saw small bakeries, cafes, and markets that opened at 5:00 A.M. sharp and swarmed with customers by 6:00 A.M. I saw people squatting on the sidewalk in front of their hovels, brushing their teeth and spitting into the gutter. And I saw men pulling large carts loaded with feces. Where they got their load and where they were taking it puzzled me.

After Nanjing, we flew 1,000 miles to Xi'an, best known for its archaeological treasures. Here I saw the carts again and learned that they contained human feces collected from nearby homes and communal privies— toilets as we know them are absent in most Chinese dwellings. After collection, the feces are taken to disposal areas for treatment before use as fertilizer. This helps explain why the tourists and natives are told not to eat uncooked vegetables or unpeeled fruit.

During one of my runs, I encountered a group of people exercising with swords. I sped back to the hotel, grabbed a camera, and returned in time to have my picture taken with them. Having our picture made together seemed as much a treat for them as it was for me. They were the only sword-wielding exercisers I saw in China, but I did see many other physical fitness seekers doing similar rhythmic calisthenics or slow-motion gymnastics. All of these meditative movements are variations of "Tai Chi Chuan," an ancient Chinese discipline practiced by old and young alike.

The single most enlightening incident of my trip occurred in Xi'an. It began when I chanced upon a large sports complex during a run at daybreak. The gates to the complex were open and I wanted to go in, but remembering my experience with the military near Wuxi, I didn't. Luckily, a young athlete standing close by sensed my feelings and said, "Good morning. Can I help you?"

He had taught himself English and spoke it well. He claimed that the Xi'an sports complex is the biggest in the world, and I could believe it after we had toured the grounds. All of the city's athletic teams from the high-school level up—thousands of athletes—live and train there. We saw his dormitory, the building in which he coached, the basketball arena and volleyball courts, the 400-meter track, and the 70,000-seat football-soccer stadium. After several runs around the complex, we parted, agreeing to meet again that night. I suggested the lobby of my hotel; he balked at that idea, recommending that we meet instead outside the hotel gates.

When he arrived that evening, the guards would not allow him through the gates. This upset me but not him, because he knew that tourist hotels are off-limits to Chinese citizens. Undaunted by such regulation, we visited on the street, exchanging addresses and phone numbers. I gave him my T-shirt from the Tucson Marathon, and he gave me a beautiful rose-colored one that he had bought especially for me.

We met again the next morning for a run, after which he introduced me to members of his team. Then we planned a final get-together for lunch. Accordingly, he gave me specific and clear instructions, written in both Chinese and English, on how to contact him by phone once my schedule became firm. (The China International Travel Service often alters the itinerary of tourists, sometimes at the last minute.) When I decided on the meeting time and place, I asked each of our four Chinese guides for help in telephoning him. Three of them hemmed and hawed and finally refused. The fourth reluctantly agreed, but only after grilling me as to how

I had met my friend, how long I had known him, and why
I was calling him. Intermittently over a three-hour span,
I watched the guide make call after call. First he said that
I had given him the wrong number. Next, he reported that
no one by my friend's name was at the number called.
Then he stated that the number was correct but that my
friend, although contacted, could not come to the phone.
Finally, he advised me that my friend had gone to lunch
and would not be back for another hour. At that point,
time ran out for me and I had to leave Xi'an. I was
frustrated, bitter, and disappointed. I had wanted to
continue this relationship after returning to Houston. But
I realized that I probably wouldn't hear from my friend
again.

Our final stop was Beijing (Peking), the capital of
China. Parts of Beijing resemble a modern American city,
with expansive thoroughfares, separate lanes for
bicycles, broad sidewalks, a subway system, and
countless high-rise apartment buildings. The main street,
Chang'an Avenue, is majestic in its width and simplicity
and remarkable for its quietness; horn blowing is
prohibited in Beijing.

Each morning I ran through the Foreign Service
District, where traffic was restricted and pistol-toting
sentries standing at attention flanked the entrances to
most of the embassies. Other runners joined me, but
most of them were Caucasian tourists staying at the
nearby Great Wall Hotel, China's newest, largest, and
most luxurious. And, for the first time, people didn't stare
at me as I jogged by. Perhaps that reflected the
sophistication of this metropolis.

Another attempt to communicate failed here. I asked
a guide—a different one, this time—to contact a local
Chinese biophysicist whom I had known in Houston and
who had visited in my home. I knew he was expecting my

call and gave his name and business phone number, written in both Chinese and English, to the guide. (Home phones are essentially nonexistent in China.) After quizzing me extensively, the guide hesitatingly complied with my request. But by then I could predict the outcome—he couldn't reach my friend.

As I reflected on this episode, certain peculiarities, some previously unmentioned, now made sense to me. The locking of our hotels and their gates, the ban against Chinese subjects entering tourist hotels, the two telephone fiascoes, the routine separation of tour groups from townsfolk in restaurants, and the requirement that tourists use special currency all could have but one logical explanation: despite its facade, the Chinese government *still* thwarts foreigners who try to establish ties with the Chinese people.

The Great Wall is a two-hour bus ride from Beijing. Tourists wishing to climb the Great Wall have two choices: an easy, gradual, even-surfaced ascent or a more difficult, steep, bumpy route. Knowing that every runner would love to trade places with me, I charge up the steeper route, running when the footing and grade permit. I continue beyond the point where tourists are advised to stop. There, on a largely decayed portion of the Great Wall, at the peak of the highest mountain in sight, I stand on top of the world. It is a great end to a glorious trip.

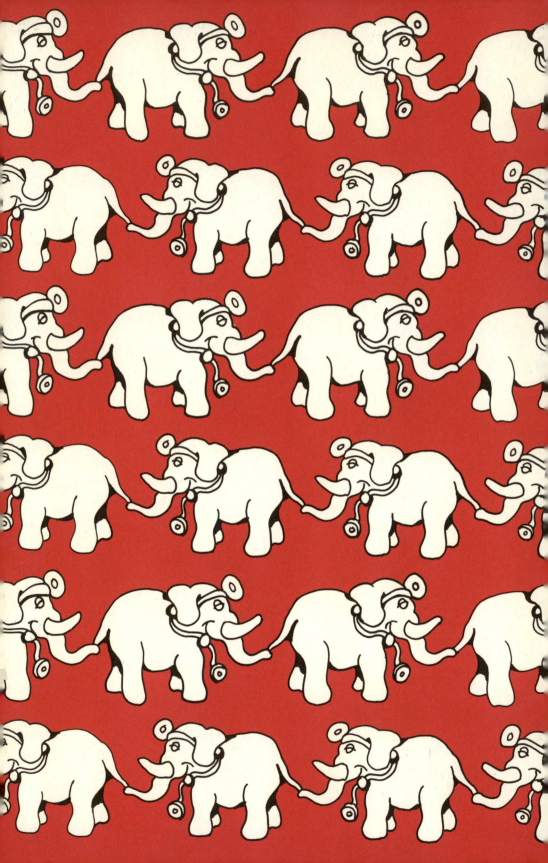